GUT HEALTH RESET

AN EASY 4-WEEK PLAN TO HELP BEGINNERS RESTORE THEIR MIND AND MICROBIOME, LOSE WEIGHT, AND RELIEVE ANXIETY

KARA HOLMES

respectfully sensitive to your individual needs. Consult your physician before making any drastic dietary changes or adding in herbs, supplements, or changing medication. The purpose of this book is not to replace medical advice or counsel of medical professionals for specific needs and circumstances.

National Eating Disorders Association Support Line:

Call: 1-800-931-2237

Text: 1-800-931-2237

National Suicide Prevention Hotline:

Text or dial: 988

Full Phone Number: 1-800-273-8255

I want to say a special thank you to Matt Jones, Janet, David, Anna, Lori, Matthew, Marrion, Leslie, Biola, Delara, Karen, Kellie, Zhen, and Karman. Thank you for supporting me with wisdom and in prayer.

Thank you, Lord for providing the resources to help this book become published. I pray that everyone who reads this receives wisdom and healing according to their unique needs.

TO THANK YOU FOR YOUR PURCHASE

Along with this book, I'm giving you **two free gifts** to support your gut healing journey:

My **Gut Healing Food, and Recipes E-Book** and **Gut Healing Herbs & Supplements Cheat Sheet!**

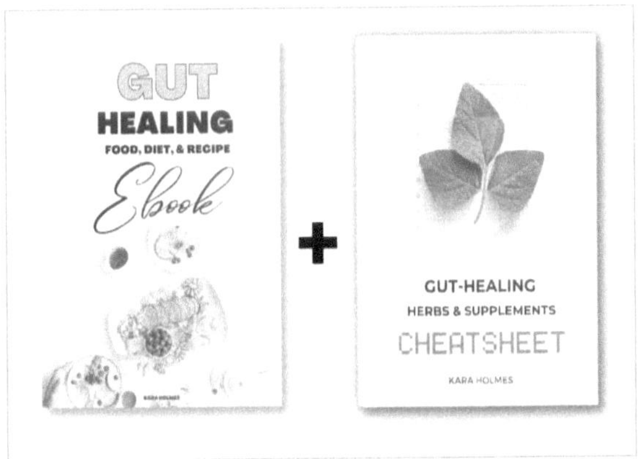

Scan the QR code to get your copy. Don't miss your chance to get:

- **Worksheets** to help you implement new habits and track your progress.
- **The Beginner's Guide to Gut-Healing Herbs and Supplements,** which will answer all your remaining questions about supplementing for gut health.
- **Over twenty additional gut-friendly recipes,** including comfort food, coffee, and desserts.
- A comprehensive, **gut-healthy grocery list.**
- A **color PDF** of the Gut Healing Plan that you can print out.
- A list of **clever, gut-healthy food and snack swaps.**

URL: https://vitalitycoaching.org/guthealthresetbonuses/

INTRODUCTION

In 2007, I developed an eating disorder that uprooted my entire life. I'd just turned sixteen and had started my first job at a fast-food restaurant. Getting a job was an important milestone in my life, one that came with more responsibility, and I wanted to be successful at it. However, I also wanted to be beautiful, approved of, and, most of all, loved. But how can you stay beautiful—that is, "thin," according to society's harsh standards—when you're working around food all the time? I'd seen other people working around food all the time and how their weight crept up over the years, and they were not happy. Before that could happen to me, I made a decision I would forever regret: I began throwing up my food to prevent myself from gaining weight. At first, I told myself I could stop whenever I wanted, even though I knew deep down that this was a lie.

Fast-forward to my early twenties, and I continued to engage in disordered eating behaviors. But now, I began using them as a method to not only prevent weight gain but also to de-stress from my classes and coursework as a nursing student. On days I didn't have class, I would wake up at 3:00 a.m. to go my part-time job as a phlebotomist at the county hospital in downtown Minneapolis. Of course, being in my early twenties, I burned the candle at both ends in an attempt to have a social life, sometimes staying up until 1:00 a.m. I was spinning out of control, and I didn't even know it. I pushed myself, telling myself things like "Everyone has to work this hard at some point in their lives. I'll take care of my health after I graduate from school." I felt as though my credibility as an emerging young woman hinged on my ability to support myself, be successful, and just be seen as a reliable, good person whom others wanted to be around. I graduated within four years, and I was able to get a job the summer after graduation. But, despite my hard work and efforts to control my health, things continued to get worse.

Even though I had a pulse and could go to my job, have relationships, and eat food, I was not truly living. I was going through the motions, and this eventually began to catch up to me.

The problems started gradually. First, I started gaining weight without eating more food. My response? Move more, eat less. I thought that I must have somehow become undisciplined and that I needed to work harder at losing weight. Through highly restrictive dieting, I managed to drop some weight. But then it came back, and then some. I began experiencing cravings and low energy that gradually became a cheap version of what I thought to be "normal" living. I'm sure you've heard countless stories like this, or perhaps you've experienced this vicious cycle firsthand.

Next, I began feeling more anxious about, well, everything. I visited my primary doctor because, along with having anxiety, I was feeling depressed. She prescribed me an antidepressant. It worked for a few months, but then I started slipping back into darkness. I would go to work, come home, watch TV, and repeat. On my days off, I would diligently exercise and do my best to eat well. I opted for eating a moderate amount of carbs and as little fat as possible, but I became confused when I couldn't maintain this rhythm of what I understood to be healthy eating. I fell into binge-eating cycles for days on end that often overlapped with drinking more alcohol than I knew I probably should. Eventually, red, rashy patches began appearing on my neck and face. Was this an allergy? It was physically painful to turn my head, and it was mentally painful to be seen. I grew impatient for answers as I scheduled and attended doctor's appointments only to walk out of each visit with negative skin and blood test results and no new answers. By now, I was stressed that I hadn't managed to figure this out. I frantically looked to elimination diets and steroids as the most viable solution. The steroids helped, but I knew they were not a long-term solution. The elimination diet was restrictive, and I couldn't maintain it with my history of disordered eating. I slowly began to accept that this was just life and I had better get used to it.

Fast-forward to 2018, when my life changed forever. A concerned friend mentioned that perhaps I should look into gut health, suggesting that it could help my skin. I had previously heard about how important the gut was to a person's overall health, but I had never paid much attention. However, by now, I was open to any and all solutions, because my everyday life was miserable.

I began looking into gut health and how it might be able to help me improve my skin and overall health. What I discovered was that the health of our gut is closely linked with the health of everything else. I could type any disease or symptom and "gut health" in the internet search bar and multiple articles, research studies, and videos would pop up. Needless to say, my curiosity had been piqued. I excitedly contacted my friend, who was also a health and wellness coach, for her recommendations on what she thought I should do to work on my gut health. We discussed several dietary and supplement ideas I could try that worked well for others, and I formulated a plan for myself based on our conversation.

Over the next six weeks, I watched miracle after miracle unfold. Years of chronic bloating disappeared. Gone. I hadn't even known how bloated I was. My skin cleared up. Moreover, my thoughts cleared, like clouds disappearing after a gloomy day. Had someone untied a blindfold that had been over my eyes?

Within that same six-week period, I forgot about my eating disorder, which was perhaps the greatest miracle I experienced. I began the journey of losing thirty pounds of weight that had been clinging to my body during the years of my bad gut and systemic inflammation. As I quickly learned, reducing inflammation and healing my gut was the answer to nearly all of my issues. Before I began to heal my gut and take care of myself differently, I felt swollen and uncomfortable but didn't have the awareness to label it as inflammation. Since the tests that were performed for systemic inflammation were not attuned to the status of my gut microbiome, I always went home with negative test results.

You've likely picked up this book because you or someone close to you is struggling with their health in some way. Are you battling painful bloating, heartburn, constipation, diarrhea, brain fog, debilitating anxiety, or an inability to lose weight despite doing everything correctly? Perhaps you've only got a few of these symptoms, or you're dealing with all of the above. I'm willing to bet you've become so frustrated that you've looked up your symptoms on Google. Perhaps you've even gone to your doctor and they've done some tests but told you, "Good news—everything came back normal!" At this point, you might have been thinking, *Am I crazy? I'm not making this up!*

I'm here to tell you that no, you're not crazy, and you're not alone either. I know how hopeless and frustrating it feels to have your doctor send you on your way with your "normal" test results when you've never felt further from normal. The Western medical system has this way of saying "you're fine" or "you're just anxious" when you feel you're nothing short of spiraling out of control health-wise. You're no longer living your best life, and no, everything's *not* fine.

As an ex-bedside RN, I believe that modern medicine is incredible and has a time and place. But from my vantage point, I can see that the infrastructure of Western medicine is a business. Unfortunately, I'm no longer certain it's the business of getting you well. What Western medicine does not tell you is that certain types of chronic conditions are manageable and some reversible by healing the underlying root cause of the issue. So, if you're curious about how you might do this in your own life and you're no longer satisfied with being sent straight to the pharmacy to get your new pill, good! I believe in a diet that doesn't come with a compounding interest agreement, gradually compounding and increasing over the years until one day your doctor tells you that you've got high blood pressure, diabetes, and dangerously high cholesterol and you need insulin and a statin. We've been sold a lie about what it means to be healthy and taught to listen to the doctor and not question anything. The problem? No one is getting better, and this needs to stop.

My first goal with this book is to serve you by revealing the true power our gut has over our entire well-being and to do so in an approachable way. Far too often, healing the gut becomes over-complicated and is explained in a way that discourages even the most intelligent people from taking the necessary steps. If I'm successful in this, I'll have met my second goal, which is to invoke enough enthusiasm inside of you to act with the information you have in your hands, begin the important journey of healing your own gut, and witness the improvement in your health that you desire. Nurturing your gut has the ability to improve your daily mood, restore your body's ability to lose unneeded weight, help you manage anxiety, and even restore libido. Furthermore, healing your gut can extend beyond yourself and can positively impact your relationships with those around you.

What is it worth to you to enjoy life feeling better than you have in years? Feeling healthy, young, and energetic is something all of us can experience. Let's discover how gut health can help with all of that, as well as much more.

You don't need to be a health expert to understand how to have a healthy gut. The information presented in this book will help you solve your stomach pain, bloating, mental health, and weight loss difficulties, and it will provide knowledge you can use to stay healthy for the rest of your life. Imagine yourself thirty years from now feeling young, healthy, and energetic. Visualize yourself feeling thankful and relieved you made some simple changes to course correct in your health journey. Now, bring yourself back to this moment. If you start now, you'll feel the difference sooner. It's never too early or too late to put your health first.

1

WHY IS THE GUT IMPORTANT?

You may have heard the saying "All disease begins in the gut," which was first stated by Hippocrates, who is known as the father of modern medicine. It's a powerful statement, but still somewhat vague. *What does that mean to me?* you might be thinking. Let's dig deeper.

When I was in school for my nursing degree, I never read a single paragraph about the gut microbiome in the textbooks for my general health, biology, or anatomy and physiology classes. If gut health is so important, why was there no training, intro, or quick blurb about it?

Well, medical textbooks and training programs are all evidence-based because treatment must be based on proof. Proper studies around the gut microbiome began getting conducted and published around the year 2000. Today, over fifty thousand studies on gut health exist. What this number of studies reveals is that there is much to uncover in the realm of gut health and that the gut is gaining recognition as a critical part of our health and wellness. The other exciting aspect of these studies is that there is now proof that healing the gut is a cornerstone to our ultimate well-being.

It wasn't until I went through my health crisis in 2017 that I took an honest look at the status of my gut health and how it was possibly playing a massive role in my mysterious condition. My eye-opening experience of healing my gut and then watching my whole life transform influences how I guide my clients now. For clients who come to me struggling with blood sugar imbalances and binge-eating, physical nourishment and the status of the gut microbiome are the first things we review together.

Gut health is defined by the quality of the digestive tissues and microbiome. Gut health refers to the physical state and physiologic function of the many parts of the gastrointestinal tract.[1] The human body has a microbiome made up of bacteria, viruses, and microbes that reside in and on the body. More than one hundred trillion microbial organisms live inside the gut, which is way more than the thirty to forty trillion cells of the average human adult. [2] So, the microorganisms that live in our gut outnumber the cells of our entire system by three times! Going on to say that the gut microbiome has the potential to impact our health is an understatement. These tiny organisms help by:

- educating the immune system to protect against harmful bacteria and viruses;[3]
- converting vitamin K1 into K2, which supports healthy bone structure;[4]
- creating vitamin B12 – bacteria have enzymes that make it, which is something plants can't do;[5]
- and supporting the growth of healthy intestinal tissue.

UNDERSTANDING **How the Gut Can Become Unhealthy**

The gut microbiome communicates with and impacts the health of our body and vice versa, meaning our gut health can suffer and become unhealthy due to other issues within our body. One of the most common causes behind an unhealthy gut is dysbiosis. In dysbiosis, the microbial population is altered in an unhelpful way—bacteria levels are too high, the types of good bacteria are outnumbered, etc.— which causes a ripple effect of issues.[6] Because the gut and the immune system have such an intertwined relationship, an unhealthy gut affects our defense and invader-recognition system.

When I was dealing with my health issues, such as my rashy skin, looking after my gut didn't occur to me because I couldn't visualize the inside of my body. However, we notice if our skin, hair, or teeth have changed, and we're quick to do something about it because it's right in our face! Pun intended.

Not only will healing the gut tissue and microbiome support improved digestion and gastrointestinal health, you'll notice less acne, better energy and sleep quality, and improved mental health.

There's also a high possibility that you're reading this book because you're already experiencing symptoms, illness, frustrations, and ailments, and you're looking for your answer.

You might be experiencing digestive problems, brain fog, or bloating that interfere with your daily life. Maybe you've been in a never-ending struggle of persistent weight gain despite caloric restriction and exercise programs. We'll cover why this happens in chapter 11. You might even be battling severe mental health issues like increased anxiety, depression, or panic attacks. It's very possible that these issues indicate gut dysbiosis and your microbiome needs support.[7] [8] Symptoms of gut dysbiosis include[9]:

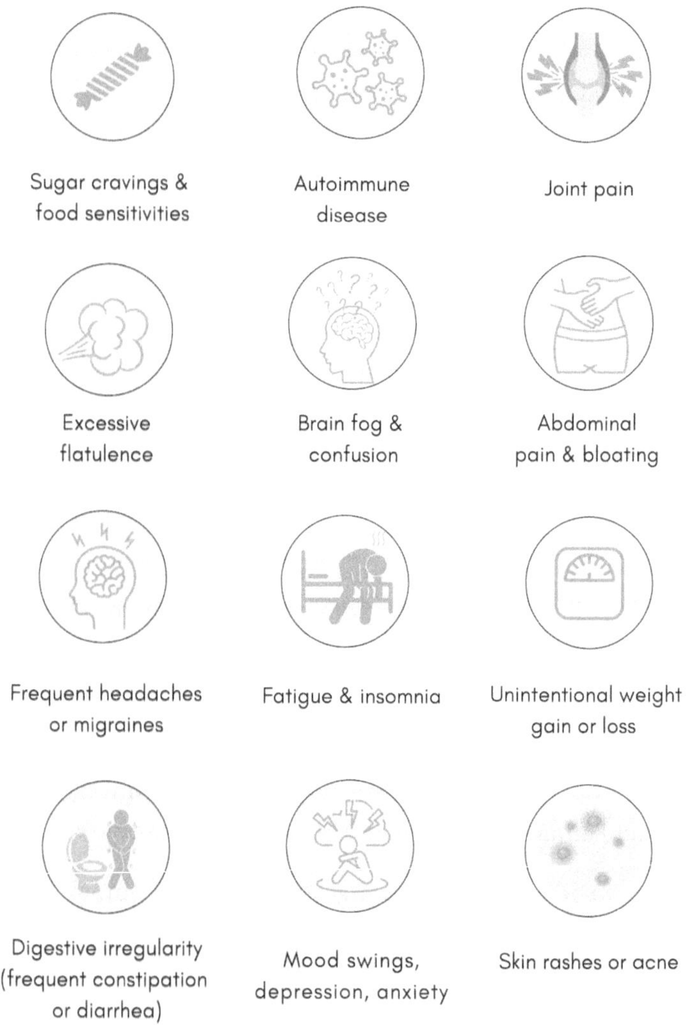

Figure 1

There are many issues that can cause dysbiosis in our system, but thankfully the road to recovery for each one is similar. The following chapters will help you gain a deeper understanding of the reasons your gut health can go downhill and what you can do to turn things around.

First, let's figure out the status of your gut. Take the following self-assessment quiz to get an idea of where you're currently at with your gut health.

Remember to consult your physician before making any drastic dietary changes, adding in herbs and supplements, or changing medication.

Gut Health Status Awareness Quiz

Instructions: Record your answers for questions 1-10 below. Write your answers down on a separate sheet of paper or on page 3 of the bonus PDF. Then head to the next page for your results.

1. Do you get an upset stomach, acid reflux, heartburn, or bloating?

Rarely / Never - 0   Sometimes - 1   Often - 2

2. Do you feel tired, exhausted, or fatigued?

Rarely / Never - 0   Sometimes - 1   Often - 2

3. Do you have food intolerances (symptoms of gas, abdominal pain, diarrhea, nausea)?

Rarely / Never - 0   Sometimes - 1   Often - 2

4. Do you have intense sugar cravings?

Rarely / Never - 0   Sometimes - 1   Often - 2

5. Do you struggle with sleep (insomnia, etc)?

Rarely / Never - 0   Sometimes - 1   Often - 2

6. Do you feel anxious or depressed?

Rarely / Never - 0   Sometimes - 1   Often - 2

7. Do you have autoimmune disease?

No - 0   Yes - 2

8. Do you have headaches or migraines?

Rarely / Never - 0   Sometimes - 1   Often - 2

9. Do you have skin issues (acne, rash)?

Rarely / Never - 0   Sometimes - 1   Often - 2

10. Have you been gaining or losing weight unintentionally or had difficulty changing your weight?

Rarely / Never - 0   Sometimes - 1   Often - 2

Figure 2

Scoring

Add up the numbers from each answer for a grand total and see which range you fall under.

0-5 =

Looking good! Experiment with adding in gut-healthy lifestyle practices outlined in this book to see if you can add more quality of life.

6-12 =

Looks like there's some room for improvement! A probiotic might be helpful, along with gut-healthy lifestyle modifications and following the plan in this book.

13-20=

Your gut health is in need of attention. It would be wise to be tested for SIBO and food intolerances and follow the gut-healing protocol outlined in this book based on the findings.

Figure 3

KEY TAKEAWAYS:

- The gut microbiome is composed of trillions of bacteria, and they help produce vitamins, support our immune system, and communicate with our brain.
- Gut dysbiosis refers to a higher population of bad bacteria microbes compared to good ones. Healing your gut involves reducing bad bacteria and repopulating the helpful ones.

2

—————

LOOKING AT THE INSIDE: DIGESTIVE SYSTEM 101

During my years as a bedside nurse, I saw a variety of digestive emergencies in the ICU. These experiences motivated me to learn how to take care of my digestive system and to teach others how to do the same. Many of the patients admitted for excruciating abdominal pain were later diagnosed with an infection somewhere in their gastrointestinal (GI) tract. When someone was diagnosed with these gastrointestinal infections, I knew the gut microbiome was playing a role. On a heartbreaking occasion, a patient would pass away from an infection that lead to sepsis, which is an extreme systemic response to an infection that damages the body's organs. Each time, I couldn't shake the feeling that there was something that could have been done before they reached the point of needing sedation and a breathing tube to possibly make it through. Then what? Would they continue to be better off after all of these extreme measures to save their life, or would they need to come back to the hospital because no lifestyle changes had been made?

The truth is, when we understand what happens inside our body and what bothers it, we can appreciate the lasting impact of small, healthy decisions around food and lifestyle. The journeys to wellness or illness have something in common: they are a result of repeated decisions, or habits, that we make every day. We make daily decisions about what we eat or drink and how much we sleep. You have the power to make consistent choices that may save your life one day. Small choices—such as picking the natural, non-glycemic sweetener instead of sugar when baking or skipping the inflammatory drive-through food to instead pick up ingredients to make burgers at home with olive oil and grass-fed meat—add up over time. Without perspective, it's easy to under-appreciate the power that the small, consistent choices we make with our food and lifestyle have on our health, starting from the inside out. Speaking of the inside, let's take a look.

A Look at the Inside: Digestive System Overview

The digestive system comprises the mouth, salivary glands, pharynx (throat), esophagus, stomach, liver, gallbladder, pancreas, small intestine, large intestine, rectum, and anus. Food begins being broken down for use in the body at the very beginning of the digestive system: the mouth. The job of the mouth and the salivary glands is to break food down and make it easier to digest, using enzymes in the saliva. The food then travels down the esophagus and through the lower esophageal sphincter, which then shuts, acting as a door to prevent food from coming back up. The esophagus is the path to the stomach, which contains low-pH hydrochloric acid for digesting and breaking down food into the smallest form possible before it journeys to the small intestine. The esophagus and stomach are made of smooth muscle tissue that is controlled by the autonomic nervous system through the parasympathetic division. In addition to helping our heart to beat and lungs to breath without conscious effort, this part of our nervous system sends signals to the enteric nervous system pathway, which activates the digestive system. In simpler terms, this means that digestion is automatic, and we don't have to think about it. To help break down and prepare food for the process of nutrient absorption in the small intestines, the liver and gallbladder release bile, and the pancreas releases enzymes as food exits the stomach.

The small intestine helps absorb the nutrients from food breakdown into our bloodstream. The enteric branch of the parasympathetic nervous system activates the migrating motor complex (MMC) to help propel food along the small intestine. From there, every tiny molecule that can be used by the body is shuttled away for a specific purpose, and the rest moves along to be eliminated as waste. Then as the blood flows through the body, it filters through the liver. The liver creates cholesterol molecules and proteins that help carry fats through the body so we can use them for energy, hormone production, or storage. After the digested food enters the small intestine, it passes through the twenty-two-foot-long large intestine, which is the passage to the colon. As the digested food enters the large intestine, it's drained of water and formed into stool before being eliminated from the body through the rectum.

Digestive System Anatomy
Mouth
Tongue
Esophagus
Stomach
Liver
Pancreas
Gallbladder
Small Intestine
(includes duodenum,
jejunum, ileum)
Large Intestine (Colon)
Appendix
Sigmoid Colon
Rectum

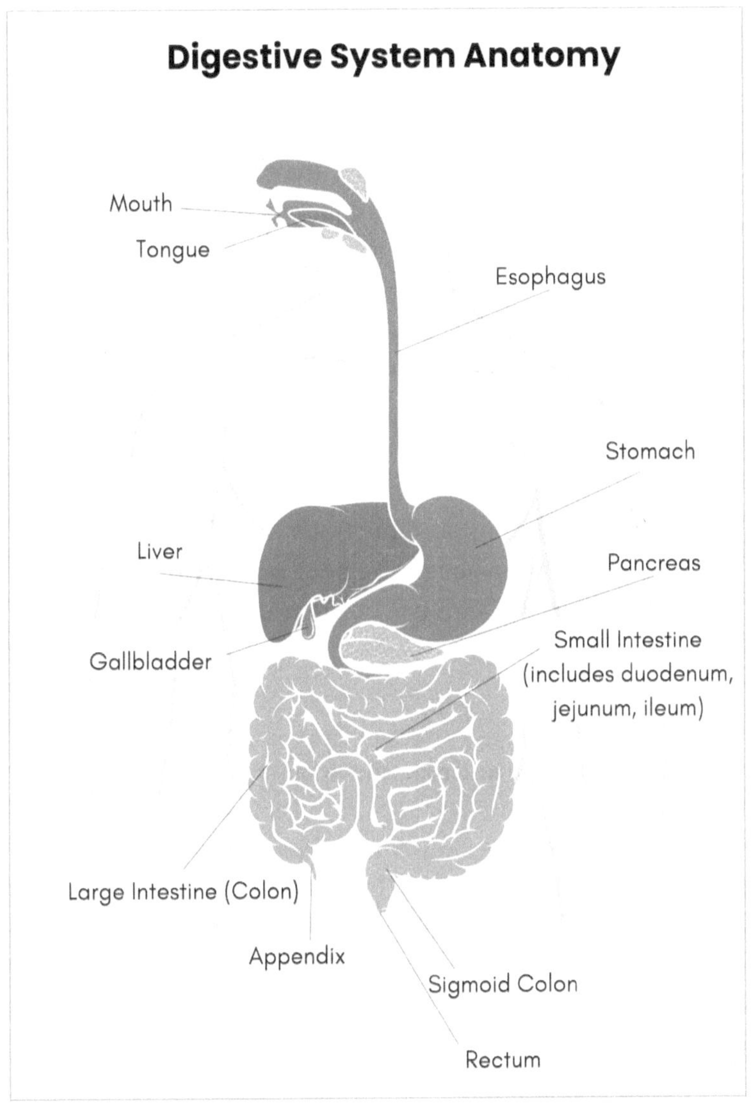

Figure 4

Is My Digestive Pattern Healthy?

Digestive patterns vary from person to person. Some have a bowel movement daily, and others twice a week. Bowel patterns don't always stay the same either; they can change based on stress and anxiety levels, physical activity, hydration, food choices, and eating habits. If it's been longer than three days between bowel movements, it's getting to be too long, and it becomes more difficult to pass the stool. Constipation happens as bowel movements become less frequent and more difficult to pass. With diarrhea, it's the opposite problem, as stools are too loose, watery, and frequent. Diarrhea can cause dehydration and electrolyte imbalances. Both constipation and diarrhea can be influenced by chronic illness, emotional distress, certain foods, medications, infections, or poor gut health. Only a small percentage of people with constipation have a serious medical condition.[1]

Signs of a happy gut and digestive system:

- One to three bowel movements daily
- Infrequent bloating (or only after a meal)
- Infrequent flatulence
- Lack of heartburn
- Hunger in the mornings (upon waking or soon after)
- Stable mood
- Stable energy level
- Clear, healthy, even glowing skin
- Stool passes easily, quickly eliminated when urge arrives
- Continence (no uncontrolled emptying of bowels)
- Infrequent diarrhea and constipation
- No abdominal pain or stomach aches

- No hemorrhoids
- No blood or undigested food in stool

SIGNS of an unhappy digestive system in need of attention and healing are the exact opposites of this list. The more symptoms you have and the more frequently they happen, the more dysregulated your digestive system could be. Seeking your doctor's opinion and taking recommended testing is a helpful first step. In chapter 10, we'll go over natural strategies and remedies to help improve your gut and digestive health. Not sure where you land on the spectrum regarding bowel activity?

- Constipation — Solid, hard, rock-like stool shaped like pellets or formed into a log. Difficult and sometimes painful to pass.
- Regular — Solid, log-like, slightly softer stool, sometimes pieces with smooth edges or some cracks on the surface. Easy and somewhat effortless to pass.
- Diarrhea — Loose, ragged, very soft, fluffy edge stool to watery, unformed, and liquid.

WARNING Signs to Never Ignore

Occasional digestive pain and bloating that occur due to breaking down food is normal, but there are some signs of digestive health you should never ignore. Seek medical attention right away if you experience any of the following.

- Having blood in your stool or throwing up blood. Blood in either stool or vomit is a sign of internal bleeding. Sometimes, people develop hemorrhoids, which are enlarged and painful blood vessels in the rectum. These can burst and bleed, and you likely won't be able to tell the difference between a hemorrhoid bleeding and deeper gastrointestinal bleeding without medical help.

- Feeling severe pain anywhere in your abdomen that doesn't go away. This pain may feel dull or sharp like stabbing or cramping.
- Seeing a yellow appearance to the skin. This is a sign that your liver health needs to be checked.
- Going longer than two weeks without a bowel movement.[2]
- Feeling like something is blocking your stool from coming out or feeling any bulging or protrusion through the vaginal canal.

<u>KEY TAKEAWAYS:</u>

- The status of the digestive system can impact the gut microbiome, and vice versa.
- You can get an idea of how happy your digestive system and gut are by noting your digestive patterns, mood, energy levels, and frequency of bloating.

3

DO YOU HAVE A HIGHER RISK OF
GUT DYSBIOSIS?

In my twenties, I went through seven years of gaining weight no matter what I did. I felt confused and frustrated, as I had an active job and exercised five days a week for thirty to sixty minutes. My reaction to the mysterious weight gain was usually putting myself on an extremely low-calorie, low-fat diet. Sometimes I would see results, but I was never able to sustain that level of restrictive eating for longer than one to two weeks. When I became exhausted from crash dieting, I would try to clean up my diet to keep the weight loss going. I always thought I needed to break through a plateau to keep losing weight because I still had more to lose. How could it be so hard? The fitness influencers made it look easy. I thought if they could do it, so could I. My clean-eating strategy looked like broccoli, salad, chicken, fish, beans, no bread, no sugar, low on calories, and low on fat. I even drank a superfood shake every day. I always thought, *This is it, I've figured it out this time.* It should have been a red flag that my binge-eating and purging patterns were very active during this time as well, but I didn't connect my restrictive food choices with my uncontrollable urge to binge on the foods I never let myself eat. Despite my best efforts of intense exercising and restrictive eating plans, the weight continued to pile on. I was bloated and constipated half the time or more. As I ventured further into my twenties, I began to think this was my "normal." How wrong I was!

Does any of this sound familiar? Unfortunately, many people find themselves in this situation and may even live like this for decades. The truth is that weight loss is not as simple as a calories in–calories out equation, not for a stressed-out body with a disrupted gut microbiome.

It's good to be eager to get to a healthier state and work toward a weight where you feel your best. However, before starting an eating plan with a calorie deficit and intense exercise regimen, you should take a good look at the state of your body. I spent too many years in misery by not understanding the basics of healing the gut and restoring disordered eating patterns to a more balanced method. This chapter will clarify lifestyle and risk factors for poor gut health and the level of stress and inflammation on the inside.

Risk Factors for Leaky Gut and Gut Dysbiosis

We discussed poor gut health symptoms in the last chapter, but did you know that certain lifestyle risk factors can predispose you to a leaky gut?

THESE RISK FACTORS ARE:

Risk Factors for Gut Dysbiosis and Poor Gut Health

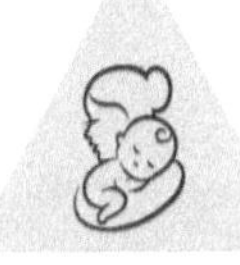

Birth Route

(i.e. Being born via C-section as a baby vs. vaginally)

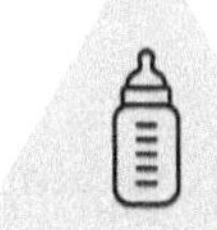

Infant Nutrition

(i.e. primarily formula-fed vs breastmilk as a baby

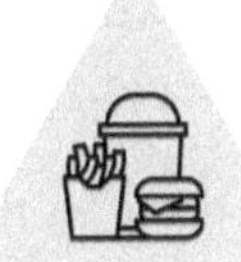

Diet

(i.e. diet high In refined carbohydrates, seed oils, alcohol, and sugars)

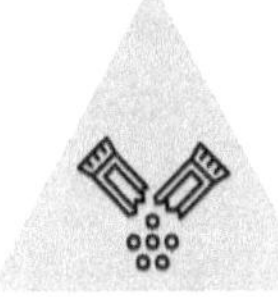

Artificial Sweeteners

(i.e. Drinking diet sodas sweetened with aspartame or sucralose)

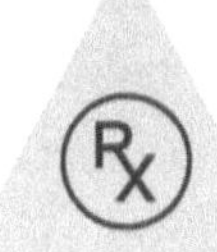

Certain Medications

(i.e. oral contraceptives, antibiotics, antacids)

Toxin & Irritant Exposure

(i.e. microplastics, pesticides, herbicides)

Chronic Stress

(i.e. caregiver burnout, demanding job, relationship turmoil)

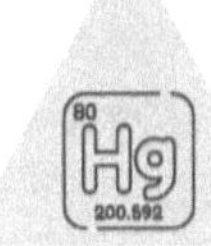

Heavy Metal Toxicity

(i.e. lead, mercury, and arsenic poisnoning)

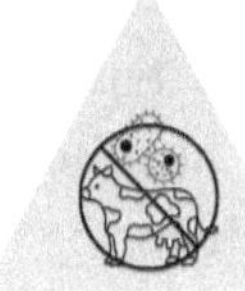

Sterile Environment

(i.e. lack of exposure to dirt and animals at a young age)

Figure 5

<u>Cesarean Birth</u> and Formula

When I first learned our gut microbiome is shaped from the minute we're born and influenced by our method of feeding, I was beside myself. There is evidence to support that babies delivered via cesarean route follow abnormal patterns of gut microbial development, as a baby born by cesarean section is not being exposed to their mother's vaginal flora as they come into the world.[1]

A study done in the United Kingdom monitored 596 babies as they were born. Of these babies, 314 were delivered vaginally and the other 282 were delivered by C-section. Data regarding the babies' microbial profile in their digestive systems at four, seven, and twenty-one days after birth.[2] The babies' gut microbes were cultured from fecal samples. The researchers made a shocking discovery: babies born via C-section were lacking in strains of symbiotic bacteria. Instead, these babies' microbiomes had a population of bacteria that resembled bacteria colonized in the hospital, namely klebsiella and ente-rococcus. These strains of bacteria can infect patients when they go to the hospital and later cause problems. Many of these strains are antibiotic-resistant. It is estimated that one in thirty-one patients admitted to the hospital will acquire an infection from this type of opportunistic bacteria. It's a big problem, costing healthcare facilities over $24 billion in the United States alone.[3]

What influence does this difference in gut microbiome composition look like in these children as they age? Studies investigating the control of diseases have suggested that C-section babies have a higher risk for asthma and obesity as they age. At nine months of age, babies born via C-section have lower than optimal levels of a bacteria strain called bacteroides in their gut, which can positively impact the immune system and help decrease inflammation.

In addition, mothers who have a C-section receive antibiotics that can cross the placenta and go to the baby. As the baby drinks breastmilk, they are exposed to additional antibiotics inside the mother's milk.

Infant Formula

Babies fed breastmilk during their first three years may have improved immune system functioning and may be less susceptible to allergies as they grow up. During the first seven to ten days of the baby's life, the mother's milk delivers important lactic acid bacterium called bifidobacterium.[4] Lactic acid bacteria coat the small and large intestines and protect the body from harmful bacteria that try to invade the body. Therefore, breastmilk has a significant role in helping the immune system from the first week of life and promotes a healthy bacterial population early on.

It may surprise you to learn that humans used to eat dirt, as a supplement of sorts, due to the gastrointestinal benefits it provides.[5] Exposure to the microbes in our environment from dirt, animals, animal dander, and more has even been shown to protect against conditions like asthma by training our immune systems from an early age.[6]

Highly Refined Carbohydrates and Sugar

The Western diet, or the standard American diet, is high in harmful fats, super-refined carbohydrates, and sugar. It is also deficient in plant fiber. These elements combined create a poor effect on health that contributes to insulin resistance, higher blood sugar levels, heart disease, and chronic low-grade inflammation. What is the link between sugary and highly refined foods and our gut? The gut microbiome responds to what we eat. Many foods packaged in boxes, freezer meals, and plastic wraps have components our bodies can't recognize, such as preservatives, texturizers, and artificial coloring, which don't originate in our natural environment and can therefore harm our digestive system if eaten as a predominant source of food.

Additionally, with high intake of sugar, the species of bacteria called bacteroidetes decreases.[7] The decreased level can harm us because bacteroidetes protect us from toxins and defend the gut barrier in other ways. For example, if the gut layer is not well-defended with helpful bacteria, and a thick enough layer of mucus, the epithelial cells that line the gut will be injured and the gut becomes leakier. In the following chapters, I'll teach you how to eat less refined foods and sugar without giving up sweets and foods you love.

ARTIFICIAL SWEETENERS

Although many artificial sweeteners are safe for our bodies, there are some that we should avoid. These include saccharin, acesulfame potassium, sucralose, and aspartame. In multiple studies, saccharin changed the gut microbiome in mice enough for glucose intolerance to be noticeable.[8] Acesulfame potassium, sucralose, and aspartame are artificial sweeteners frequently used in diet drinks. These sweeteners in particular are associated with obesity and higher levels of inflammation.[9] Thankfully, there are plenty of other soft drinks, some even with prebiotic fibers in them, to choose from that are created with natural and alternative sweeteners that don't cause inflammation. Some of them even support thriving gut bacteria. A full list of gut-healthy swaps for diet soda can be found in the bonus PDF (found in the front and back of this book with an easy-access QR code). Sweeteners to look for within the ingredients list are monk fruit extract and allulose. In later chapters, we'll cover more about alternative sweeteners useful for balancing blood sugar and gut health.

ALCOHOL

Drinking excessive amounts of alcohol exerts unhelpful changes in the gut microbiome, increases leaky gut, and interferes with normal functioning of the liver.[10] Impaired liver function comes from processing the alcohol, and secondarily from inflammation that comes with leaky gut and circulating bacteria and toxins. When the liver can't properly do its job, the gut is impacted. Bile is made in the liver, and the health of our gut tissue and gut microbiome rely on proper bile flow. You can begin to see how one problem impacts the other, and the damaging loop continues unless healing can take place.

MEDICATIONS

Antibiotics

Antibiotics, acid reflux medications, and non-steroidal anti-inflammatory drugs (such as ibuprofen) certainly impact the diversity of gut microbiota and essential stomach acid for digesting food. Antibiotics, particularly broad-spectrum varieties, damage the diversity and balance of the microbial community. The effects do not discriminate—changes in the bacterial community happen from short-term and long-term use of antibiotics. In some studies, antibiotic exposure has been connected to obesity and diabetes in mice. I'm not against antibiotics. I've witnessed intravenous antibiotics save the lives of patients suffering from life-threatening, blood-borne bacterial infections. I've been up against a few urinary tract infections (UTIs) myself in the past, and I was grateful that the antibiotics were given to me because I was so uncomfortable and the cranberry juice just wasn't working.

Unfortunately, your antibiotic exposure doesn't stop after completing your antibiotics course. As you may or may not know, there are also antibiotics in our food. It's estimated that over two-thirds of the antibiotics in food come from animals. It's imperative to eat antibiotic-free, hormone-free, grass-fed, and free-range animals when consuming meat products.[11] The health and composition of our gut microbiota rely on it, as does the need to reduce the massive burden of microbial-resistant bacteria that is costing the United States healthcare system billions of dollars each year.

ORAL CONTRACEPTIVES

Oral contraceptives have been gaining a reputation for their negative impact on intestinal inflammation and the development of inflammatory bowel diseases (IBD) such as Crohn's disease. Additionally, they increase leaky gut.[12] Oral contraceptives are also known to naturally decrease vitamin C, zinc, B2, B6, B12, and magnesium.[13]

PROTON PUMP INHIBITORS (PPIs)

Proton Pump Inhibitors such as pantoprazole are prescribed by doctors to treat gastroesophageal reflux disease (GERD), commonly known as acid reflux. These medications suppress acid secretion of the stomach, resulting in less acid altogether. Having adequate amounts of stomach acid is important for digesting food so the body can absorb nutrients and minerals, and killing off bacteria and parasites in our food. Oddly enough, heartburn is a symptom of having low levels of stomach acid. Impaired digestion from low stomach acid levels creates gas bubbles with stomach acid mixed in that rise up into the esophagus.[14] PPIs interfere with the gut's natural defense system and ability to have a thriving microbiome, so it's best to heal your gut and solve the root cause of acid reflux issues rather than taking these medications for life and dealing with the downstream health issues that come with.

HEAVY METALS

Every once in a while, you may hear a story about how someone who had mysterious health problems for years finally discovered it was due to heavy metal poisoning. You might wonder, how can toxic levels of heavy metals get inside the body? Well, humans and animals can become exposed to heavy metals through the soil, drinking water, polluted air, implanted bodily devices, pipes, and food.

Heavy metals naturally occur in the environment and are necessary for life, but they can over accumulate in the body and cause organ dysfunction. Serious metal ingestion over a prolonged period has even been linked with cancer. These metals change the gut microbiome. Some get excreted through the body's natural detoxification and elimination processes, and some are absorbed into the body and deposited into the organs.[15] The most common heavy metals that can cause problems are arsenic, cadmium, chromium, lead, and mercury.[16]

Arsenic, most commonly found in well water, can also be embedded in soil, fish, and shellfish. If you find yourself around coal and oil mining sites or industrial plants, be wary of high cadmium concentrations in the ground. Additionally, be careful not to eat food farmed around these sites, as cadmium contaminates the soil from burning waste products such as plastic and batteries. Cadmium contaminates the ground through the leaking of sewage into farming soil, which is then absorbed by plants that are harvested and go into the stores for people to eat. Cigarette smoke also contains cadmium. Smokers have four to five times the amount of cadmium in the blood than nonsmokers.[17] Chromium, which is found in Earth's crust and sea, has contaminated the ocean through industrial processes and manufacturing. Over-accumulation of chromium in the organs has been associated with cancer.[18] Lead is still used to manufacture car batteries, gun ammo, cable sheathing, weights, and radiation protection equipment. Exposure can occur from improper open burning and disposal of lead products or frequent contact with products containing lead without proper protective gear. Although emissions have decreased in most countries in the past forty years and water treatment has been improved to reduce lead exposure, some developing countries still manufacture paints and plastics with lead inside. The highest blood levels of lead throughout the world can be found in Latin America, the Middle East, Asia, and some parts of Eastern Europe.[19] Mercury is found in water, air, soil, fish, and seafood, and it also naturally occurs in the crust of the earth. Industrially, mercury is used in lamp factories and the production of fluorescent light bulbs. It was used in medicine until the 1920s but has since been replaced with safer compounds during manufacturing. However, it is still found in some multidose vial vaccines.[20]

Gut microbes may have a positive effect in eliminating heavy metals from the body. In one study, bacteria loaded with arsenic, lead, and cadmium related to excreted feces with higher levels of these metals, suggesting that gut microbes may help remove heavy metals once inside the gastrointestinal tract.[21]

Toxin and Irritant Exposure

Microplastics

We are all familiar with the durability of plastic. Its difficulty to break down makes it highly useful, but it poses a threat to not only our gut but our entire health. It's a nightmare, but each human takes in between fifty thousand to one-hundred-twenty thousand particles of plastic each year from the air, food, dust, bottled water, and more.[22] Bisphenol A (BPA) and phthalates are the most common plastics that cause health problems. These microplastics have been found responsible for the death of cells, some allergic reactions, and disruption of hormones resulting in cancer and interfering with fetal development. Microplastics' effect on the gut is damaging in more ways than one. These particles cause gut inflammation, damage the gut's epithelial cell layer, shrink the mucus layer protecting the lining, disturb the microbial balance, and are toxic to the immune cells surrounding the gut.[23] You can reduce your plastic exposure by switching your food containers, disposable water bottles, and plastic bags to glass or stainless-steel containers. Also, beware of nonstick cookware. These cooking pans are made with Teflon that has a layer of polytetrafluoroethylene (PTFE), which is a plastic polymer that can release toxic fumes at temperatures over 572 degrees Fahrenheit.[24] Ceramic cookware can also contain lead, so you can further reduce the toxin load on your body by using 100-percent nontoxic ceramic, glass, and enamel-coated cast-iron cookware.[25]

．　．　．

PESTICIDES

When I was a young girl, my dad assigned me to weeding duty in the garden every weekend in the summertime. I used to beg him to spray the food and soil with weed killer and pesticides so I wouldn't have to pull as many weeds. My priority was to have a chores list that was as short as possible so I could ride my bike with my neighborhood friends. Had I known the effects of these chemicals on the body, I would have never suggested it and happily pulled all those weeds! While pesticides and herbicides seem like a good idea, they can quickly get into our bodies and have harmful effects. Some of these chemicals do not even have a targeted pathway for elimination inside the body. In addition, the gut microbiome and neurotransmitter production are disturbed by the pesticide diazinon.[26] In commercial farming, diazinon pesticides are sprayed on fruit trees, flowers, berries, and vegetables.

How is our body going to get rid of foreign substances without having a pathway to neutralize and dispose of them? Our liver, our natural detoxification system, is just one of the essential organs that bear the burden of these toxins that get stuck inside our tissues and cannot escape the body.

DISORDERED EATING PATTERNS

Although not currently included in the list of risk factors, disordered eating patterns are being investigated as a contributor to gut dysbiosis.[27] The most common eating disorders are anorexia nervosa and bulimia nervosa. Severe restrictions on food and calories characterize anorexia. Bulimia involves binge-eating large quantities of food and purging afterward through over exercising, vomiting, or laxative use. To have a healthy gut microbiome, we must have diversity in the bacteria population, which becomes disrupted with eating disorders and the irregular nutrition. Beneficial bacteria that live in our gut feast on prebiotic fibers in food that we eat, mainly fibers found in fruits, vegetables, and other plant nutrients. If not eaten frequently, if purged, or if avoided all together, this deficiency will impact your gut microbiome's ability to thrive.

Furthermore, with anorexia, the body is starved, and cells and organ tissue begin to die. If this is not corrected, unfortunately, the damage can be permanent. With bulimia nervosa, the physical act of vomiting will erode the esophagus and cause bleeding and dysfunction of the esophageal sphincter. Over time, this can scar, and acid can leak backward into the esophagus, causing burning pain that most of us know as heartburn. When digestive and intestinal tissue becomes damaged, the mucus layer of the gut and the bacteria that live there are likely to be affected. Could this be why eating disorders, digestive disorders, and mental health problems often accompany each other?[28] Only research can reveal the answer.

IF YOU'VE READ through this chapter and feel uneasy, let me reassure you that this is entirely normal. Many of the risk factors we have for poor gut health are out of our control because they're in the past. Relax and know that there are changes you can make in your lifestyle that can support gut healing long-term and reap benefits that last.

It's one of the most potent acts of self-love to be able to consistently eat food that is going to help your body shift into a regenerative state and thrive. I'll venture to say that once you do this consistently, you won't want to turn back to the packaged, high sugar, and high carbohydrate foods you were eating most days. Feeling better changes you beyond the physical sensation. You will feel more energetic than you have in years, and you will begin to see your self-worth as more valuable. You'll be able to identify other areas where perhaps you haven't been choosing the best for yourself. The important part is remembering that you can't expect to make all these changes overnight. Rather than getting discouraged and avoiding making any changes all together, focus on one area or one step at a time. This month, you might stop drinking Diet Coke and swap it for a prebiotic version of cola. Next month, it could look like buying a new stainless-steel frying pan to replace the nonstick pan you currently use. It may not seem like it right away, but these one-step changes soon add up to a large list and snowball into noticeable changes in your health. Making these small, health-minded decisions can even inspire you to change other areas of your life and catch fire in your relationships, finances, and career. Metaphorically, your life can begin to resemble a blossoming garden, and the end result will be a gift to maintain.

<u>KEY TAKEAWAYS:</u>

- You have some control over your risk for gut dysbiosis (i.e. sugar and artificial sweetener intake) but other risk factors are out of your control (i.e. birth route).
- When healing your gut, focus on changing the lifestyle areas you have control over one by one.

4

UNDERSTANDING IBS, SIBO / SIFO, AND LEAKY GUT SYNDROME

In this chapter, we'll shine light on some of the most common conditions associated with gut dysbiosis—irritable bowel syndrome (IBS), small intestinal bacterial and fungal overgrowth (SIBO/SIFO), and leaky gut syndrome.

You may be thinking, *Which one do I have? I have symptoms that overlap between all of them.* It's common for more than one to be present at the same time. It can be frustrating, but the good news is the treatment of each one focuses on the same goals:

1. Correct dysbiosis by decreasing harmful bacteria and other organisms
2. Restore integrity of the gut tissue and mucosal barrier
3. Diversify helpful bacteria

Thankfully, there are things you can do that support the healing of all three.

IRRITABLE BOWEL SYNDROME (IBS)

IBS happens to be the most common digestive disorder gastroenterologists encounter among the patients they see.[1] Characterized by varying degrees of abdominal pain and changes in bowel patterns, IBS has a number of presumed causes. Some experts suspect that 80 percent or more of IBS cases are actually misdiagnosed SIBO. With IBS, quality of life suffers. Along with the digestive discomfort of bloating, gas, unpredictable bowel habits, and abdominal pain, mental health issues such as anxiety and depression can arise. The brain and the gut are in a close relationship, so it makes sense that what affects the gut also affects the brain and vice versa.[2] Because there are so many reasons and potential contributing factors to IBS, it's important to figure out the root of the issue. If you are diagnosed with IBS, it's likely your physician will assign a type to your diagnosis. An IBS-C diagnosis describes constipation symptoms accompanying IBS. IBS-D is assigned when diarrhea is a primary symptom.

Causes of Irritable Bowel Syndrome

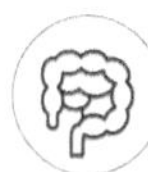

Bowel Motility Issues

- paralyzed bowel tissue
- nervous system disorders
- dysfunction of Migrating Motor Complex

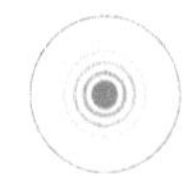

Visceral hypersensitivity

- Your organs sense pain at a lower threshold
- Also seen in disorders affecting the nervous system (i.e. fibromyalgia)

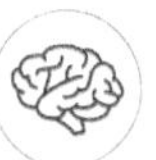

Gut-Brain Interactions

- Irritability is a response to an interaction between the gut and brain (i.e. anxiety, stress, and panic)

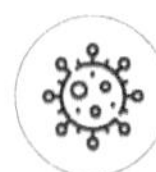

Post-Infection Reactivity

- Bowels are in a more reactive state after fighting off an infection, such as a stomach bug, Traveler's diarrhea, and more.

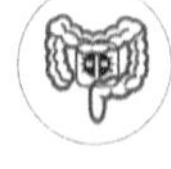

Change in the Microbiome

- The concentration and population of microbes has changed, possibly from many rounds of antibiotic therapies killing off good bacteria.

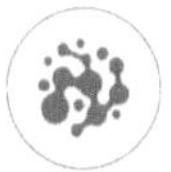

Bacterial Overgrowth

- Overgrowth of unhelpful bacteria that causes inflammation (SIBO/SIFO)

Intestinal Inflammation

- Various causes, consider Chrohn's disease and Ulcerative Colitis, acute infections such as colitis and diverticulitis,

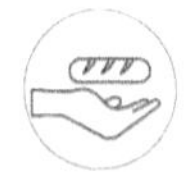

Poor Carb Absorption

- Problems absorbing carbohydrates during digestion

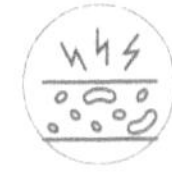

Food Sensitivities

- Body's intolerance to particular foods Irritating the bowel and continuous exposure over time can contribute to IBS.

Figure 6 - Reference: See Weaver, K. R., Melkus, G. D., & Henderson, W. A. (2017) for more information on Irritable Bowel Syndrome

Managing IBS

Sorting out IBS root causes, food triggers, or symptom relievers will not be a straightforward process, but there are some strategies to try implementing that can be supportive in symptom management and decreasing stress that we'll cover in this chapter and in chapter 5. Stress on the inside of our body will have some effect on the gut, whether you feel it or not. There's no documented cure for IBS, but considering that if it has a root cause, correcting that will provide grounds for healing you might not have expected. However, if you actually have SIBO and have an IBS misdiagnosis, you'll be pleased to read the next section because you can actually treat SIBO and experience permanent remission.

Strategies That May Help with IBS & Symptom Management

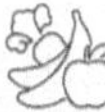

Get adequate dietary fiber from fruits, nuts, whole grains, vegetables, and psyllium husk.

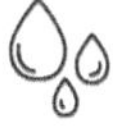

Adequate hydration. Drinking eight 8-10 oz glasses of water per day supports hydration. Tea and carbonated sodas count.

Don't smoke. Smoking irritates and stimulates the intestines and is linked with various cancers.

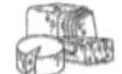

Consider trying to decrease or remove dairy. Many people with IBS have lactose intolerance. Obtain calcium through supplementation or by eating dark green vegetables.

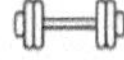

Exercise regularly. Exercise is a natural intestinal regulator and supports a healthy gut microbiome.

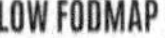

LOW FODMAP

Decrease FODMAP foods. These foods are high in carbs and fibers, can cause bloating and other symptoms.

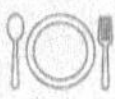

Eat smaller meals more often. Try to space meals to be 3-4 hours apart.

Relaxation techniques. Diaphragmatic breathing and other breathwork, stretching, prayer, and mindfulness may support your nervous system and IBS management.

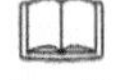

Keep a food journal. Record the foods that make you have an IBS-flareup and the circumstances around eating. (i.e. stressed out, at work, morning, evening, etc.)

Figure 7 - Reference: See Irritable bowel syndrome - Diagnosis and treatment - Mayo Clinic (2021) for more information.

Small Intestinal Bacterial and Fungal Overgrowth (SIBO/SIFO)

Small intestinal bacterial overgrowth refers to an increase in population of gut bacteria in the small intestine, possibly an imbalanced amount of unhelpful gut microbes.[3] Most of our gut bacteria live in the colon, but certain circumstances can encourage growth farther up in the intestinal tract.[4]

An overgrowth of fungi in the small intestine, often called candidiasis or "candida overgrowth," can cause issues similar to SIBO. SIBO and SIFO can be present at the same time. You can't spread SIBO to other people. In addition to causing dysbiosis, SIBO can even interfere with fat and carbohydrate absorption, resulting in diarrhea and malnutrition. The imbalance and overgrowth of certain bacteria can lead to fat-soluble vitamin deficiency—namely vitamins A, D, E, and K—as well as B12 deficiency, which can lead to nervous system damage that cannot be undone.[5] This damage can manifest as paralysis, dementia, depression, or osteoporosis. So it is imperative you don't leave SIBO alone and instead take action to correct it.

COMMONLY REPORTED Symptoms of People with SIBO/SIFO

- Bloating – Upper and lower abdominal bloating that some say resembles a "six-month pregnant belly."
- Burping and flatulence – Belching and foul-smelling, frequent gas.
- Diarrhea – Loose stool, often unpredictable. People can begin to restrict and fear many foods.
- Abdominal pain

WHAT CAUSES this increase in bacteria or fungi in the small intestine? Due to SIBO being characterized by gut dysbiosis, you'll notice many risk factors overlap.

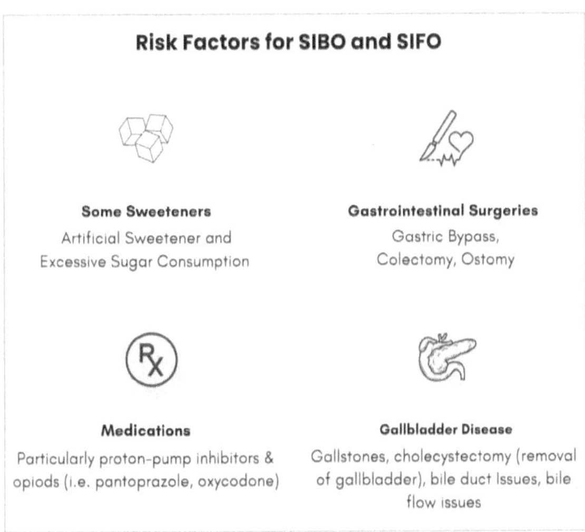

Figure 8 - Reference: See Small intestinal bacterial overgrowth (SIBO) - Symptoms and causes (2022) Mayo Clinic for more information.

GASTROINTESTINAL SURGERY

Interestingly, a large percentage of patients having undergone surgery that removes part of the stomach or bowel due to gastric bypass, cancer, trauma, or disease have higher incidences of SIBO, reporting fatigue, digestive pattern irregularity, and bloating.[6] Is this a survival response by the body in an attempt to rebalance after a significantly large portion of the gut flora disappeared along with the surgery? So far, there isn't a definitive explanation for what causes this at a cellular and tissue level.

· · ·

Dysmotility

Dysmotility, or irregular functioning of the migrating motor complex (MMC) in the body, is a risk factor for SIBO due to food spending prolonged periods in the digestive tract, which can actually cause bacteria to grow upward and therefore worsen SIBO. Bacteria are mostly supposed to be in the colon, not in the small intestine. Since bacteria feed on carbs, fiber, and sugar, the higher your diet is in them, the more bloating you can experience depending on how many bacteria are in your small intestine. This is why following blanket advice like "just eat more prebiotic foods" can get people with SIBO into trouble—prebiotic fiber feeds the good bacteria and the bad bacteria. See chapter 6 for more information about when prebiotic fiber is helpful and when it may hinder healing.

GALLBLADDER DISEASE

Another potential risk factor for SIBO is gallbladder disease or the presence of gallstones.[7] The gallbladder stores and releases bile made by the liver in order to support emulsification of fats so the pancreas can break them down for energy with enzyme action. If bile is blocked due to issues with the duct, such as in the case of gallstones, it cannot flow into the small intestine. Regular bile function is an important factor for inhibiting bacterial overgrowth in the small intestine. Taking sunflower lethicin, probiotic foods, eating bitters, and chewing food more slowly can naturally support healthy bile flow.[8] Pain in the right upper quadrant of the abdomen, yellowing of skin, and clay-colored stools can all be signs of gallbladder dysfunction.

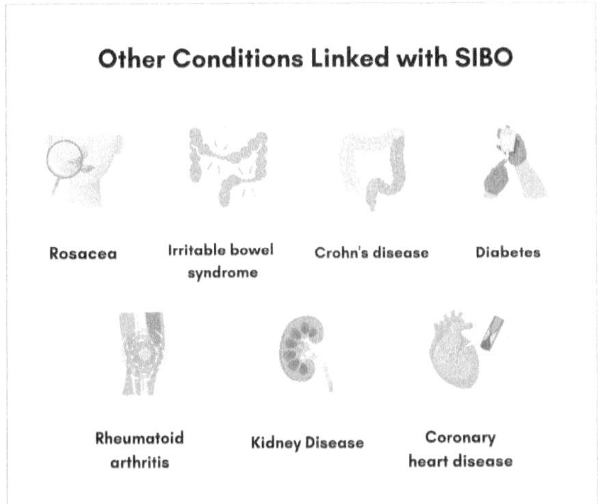

Figure 9 - References: See Weiss, E., & Katta, R. (2017) for more information on SIBO and rosacea, Huh, J. , Ruscio, M. (2022) for more information on SIBO and medical conditions, and 'Associated Diseases. (n.d.). (2022)' for more information on SIBO and associated diseases.

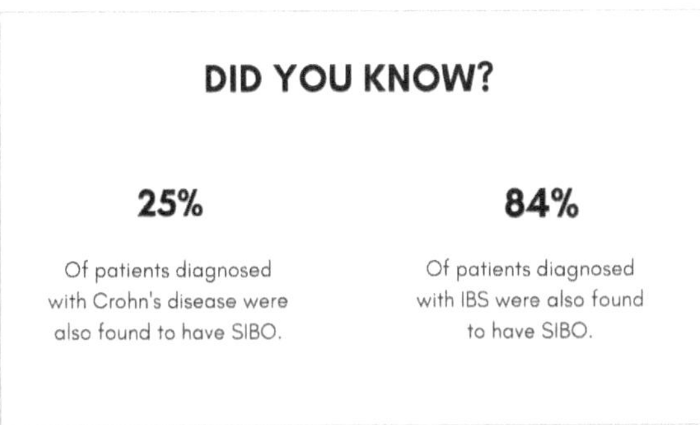

Figure 10 - Reference: See Associated Diseases. (n.d.). (2022) for more information on SIBO - Small Intestine Bacterial Overgrowth

SIBO Types

There are actually three different SIBO types: hydrogen-dominant, methane-dominant, and sulfide-dominant. SIBO classification is helpful because it enables more accurate treatment. For example, methane-dominant SIBO is often referred to as SIBO-C and is associated with archaea overgrowth. Since archaea are not bacteria, antibiotics won't effectively treat its overgrowth, and your SIBO won't go away. This is why it's important to be informed about all options available in the setting of healing SIBO, such as herbal antimicrobials, dietary changes, and probiotics.

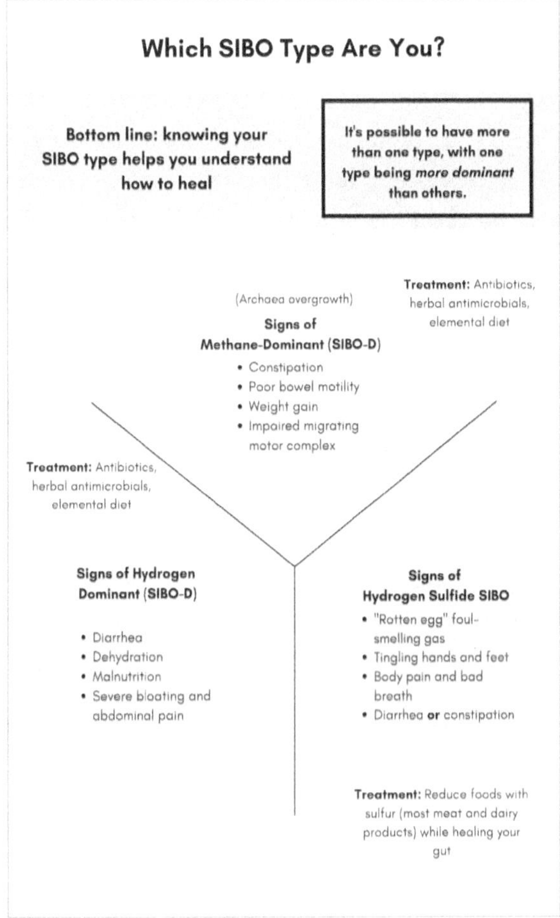

Figure 11 - Reference: See Source: Team, T. N., Saldivar, G., (2021) for more information on how to heal the 3 types of SIBO.

Effective Diagnosis and Treatments for SIBO

If you're concerned you might have SIBO, there are a few tests available to help give you answers:

- Breath tests
- Small bowel aspiration

The breath test is typically favored when assessing for SIBO because it's the easiest, least invasive option. When sugar is consumed, bacteria metabolize it and release hydrogen or methane gas. These can be detected in your breath. To take a test, you can purchase a breath test kit to have on hand, or you can go through the process of asking your doctor for help scheduling one, then paying for a one-time test. Purchasing a test kit can be a worthwhile investment if you plan to test for SIBO again in the future. After you've worked on rebalancing your gut flora by decreasing inflammation and overall bacteria in the small intestine for a couple months, you might want to check how your body has responded to the changes you made. Check the back of this book for recommended kits. Whether it's an in-clinic test or a test kit you purchase yourself, ensure the test is capable of testing for methane gas. A separate kind of organism, which are called archaea and are not classified as bacteria, can be part of SIBO and they actually consume hydrogen released from bacteria.[9] Archaea eat the hydrogen and then produce methane gas. If archaea species are part of SIBO, you can see why a hydrogen breath test could come back negative—the archaea can consume it all and then there's none left to test.

When taking a breath test, the instructions may have you consume a sugar-sweetened beverage before testing. Usually, if a test comes back with noted hydrogen within ninety minutes after taking the test, it's possible you have SIBO. Since bacteria are supposed to live in the large intestine, it should take over two hours until the food or sugar reaches that point in the process of digestion. So the early hydrogen reading suggests that sugar is reaching the bacteria farther up the GI tract and you may have an overgrowth there.

A couple of downsides of breath testing are false-positive results and how much preparation must go in beforehand. The truth is that some people digest and metabolize food differently than others, and this can be a potential issue when relying on test results to tell you if you have SIBO. Most breath tests require you to avoid antibiotics, probiotics, and other medications for up to four weeks prior. For two days before the test, you will likely be asked to eat low-carbohydrate meals in order to prepare your body and make it more sensitive to the sugar before the test.

Aspiration of the small bowel is an invasive test that requires sedation and an endoscopy of your upper small bowel. A fluid sample of your small intestine is taken, likely from the jejunum. This test tends to be the less favorable option due to the invasive nature and also due to fact that most endoscopes and colonoscopes,[10] the cameras that doctors use to look into the GI tract, measure only one to six feet long[11] and therefore cannot actually see the entire small bowel, which is twenty-two-feet long on average. With an entire seventeen feet of small bowel left unexplored,[12] this leaves a lot of room for false-negative results.[53]

MEDICATIONS, Herbs, and Supplements

Numerous antibiotics have been tested on people for eradicating SIBO, but the most effective one across fifteen studies has been Rifaximin.[13] Understandably, it's become the favorable choice for treatment of SIBO by many doctors. However, there are a few things to consider before taking this antibiotic.

- Antibiotics, including Rifaximin, kill off all bacteria indiscriminately, good and bad. If antibiotics alter gut flora and that altered gut flora causes dysbiosis in the gut, it's possible that antibiotic use may contribute to SIBO, which is a horrendous concept because that's what we're trying to fix in the first place.
- Antibiotics, including Rifaximin, have their share of side effects: diarrhea, nausea, headaches, swelling of hands and extremities, dizziness, fever, and flatulence. Having these symptoms on top of what you're already going through can be overwhelming.[14]
- The price can be restrictive for some. Currently, the retail price of thirty tablets of Rifaximin is nearly $1,700.[15] If you have insurance that covers the medication, you'll likely be spending $60 to $80 instead, which still adds up.
- Nearly half of patients will be recommended for re-treatment by their doctors at the nine-month mark because of suspected SIBO recurrence.[16] For a large portion of individuals, this treatment won't put an end to their issue.
- If you rely only on antibiotics for treatment of SIBO, you're not getting to the bottom of why the SIBO and gut dysbiosis developed in the first place. Doesn't discovering and treating the root cause of an issue in order to eliminate it sound more appealing than adding yet another pill?

THANKFULLY, herbal therapies for SIBO are recognized as being equally as effective as Rifaximin, if not more so. In one study, the herbal therapy was actually more effective in treating SIBO, having a 45 percent success rate, as more of this group's participants had a negative breath test with no relapse after treatment compared to the Rifaximin group, which only had a 34 percent success rate. Herbal preparations included in the study were FC-Cidal, Dysbiocide, and Candibactin-AR and BR.[17]

Believe it or not, garlic has potent antibacterial properties that can even be effective against helicobacter pylori (H. pylori), a bacterial infection in the stomach.[18] Many cultures have used it for centuries, even dating back over three thousand years. It's uses have varied from cancer to dysentery, and there is plenty of anecdotal evidence supporting that garlic helped people successfully treat their SIBO, as well as their IBS.[19] Curcumin, the active compound found in turmeric root, successfully reduced abdominal pain, bloating, and anxiety in patients with IBS and SIBO in a double-blind research trial.[20] Ginger and 5-hydroxytryptophan (5-HTP) have also been found to improve bowel motility and reduce the time that stool spends in the small bowel and colon.

Herbal Antibiotics That Have Promising Effects on SIBO

FC Cidal®	Dysbiocide®	Candibactin-AR®	Candibactin-BR®
Highlighted Ingredients:	**Highlighted Ingredients:**	**Used for SIFO - Highlighted Ingredients:**	**Used for SIBO - Highlighted Ingredients:**
• pau d'arco • *Equisetum arvense* (stem) • *Tinospora cordifolia* (stem)	• Dill stem • Acacia catechu stem extract • Yarrow leaf and flower extract (*achillea millefolium*)	• Lemon balm • Oregano oil • Sage • Red thyme oil	• Indian barberry root extract • Chinese rhubarb • Chinese licorice root (*glycyrrhiza uralensis*)

Honorable Mentions

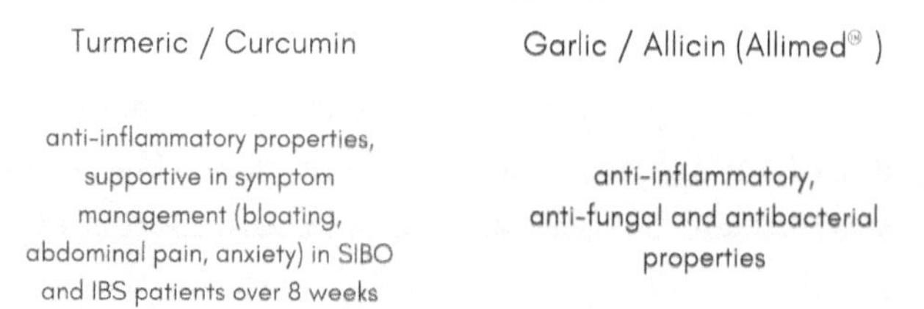

Turmeric / Curcumin	Garlic / Allicin (Allimed®)
anti-inflammatory properties, supportive in symptom management (bloating, abdominal pain, anxiety) in SIBO and IBS patients over 8 weeks	anti-inflammatory, anti-fungal and antibacterial properties

See the Resource section in the back of this book on where to find these products.

Figure 12 - References: See Chedid, V., Dhalla, S. (2014). for more information on herbal therapy compared to rifaximin in the treatment of SIBO, Ansary, J., Forbes-Hernández, T. Y. (2020) for more information on garlic uses in SIBO, and Lopresti, A. L., Smith, S. J. (2021) for more information on symptom management In SIBO and IBS with curcumin.

WHY TREAT SIBO with antibiotic medications or herbal blends? Many populations of bacteria involved in overgrowth like this are resistant to treatment due to biofilms that surround them, which resemble a bubble and act as a strong shield for bacteria. These biofilms help microbes expand and overpopulate in unhealthy amounts, requiring strong compounds to function as an artillery of sorts to break down the defense shields, allowing the microbiome to become balanced again.[21]

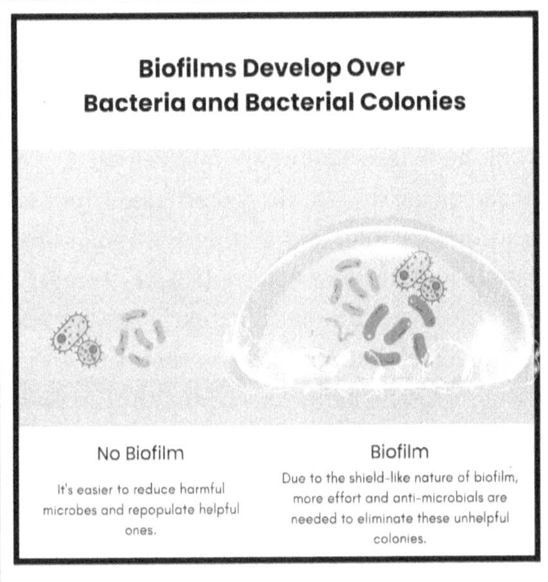

Figure 13

Food and Dietary Strategies to Reduce SIBO

In some cases of SIBO, a provider may recommend the elemental diet, which comprises liquid meals that have changed nutrients into an easily absorbable and less allergenic and inflammatory form.[22] The purpose of this is to reduce over-grown microbes but still provide nutrition to the body. The bacteria don't interact with these meals in the same way as regular food, which must be broken down in the GI tract.

. . .

ANOTHER STRATEGY that can be useful is reducing high FODMAP foods, which are foods high in starches, carbs, certain fibers, and sugar. Eating significantly less FODMAP foods will result in unhelpful bacteria being fed less, and it will be easier to bring your microbiome back into balance. We'll review this in detail in chapter 7.

It can also be beneficial to employ intermittent fasting. Eating all your meals for the day within a shortened window, 8:00 a.m. to 4:00 p.m. for example, and fasting the remaining hours of the day defines intermittent fasting (IF). IF is not a new technique, as it's been documented as early as the 1940s, when scientists discovered that it could lengthen the lives of mice.[23] Although weight loss benefits reported with IF are inconsistent, it's been proven to improve blood sugar balance and metabolic health, as well as lower type 2 diabetes, cancer, and heart disease in people.[24] When the body is allowed a fasting period with no food, the digestive system rests and has more time to repair cells and tissues. Additionally, some experts propose that the mild stress placed on the body from a fast causes cells to become more resilient and stronger, which could result in improved longevity and immunity.[25] The results repeat themselves consistently—intermittent fasting may positively benefit people struggling with obesity and type 2 diabetes because of the way it supports healing of insulin resistance and stabilizing of blood sugar response. These are also stressors that are incredibly harmful if left unchecked, and intermittent fasting can be a helpful solution to improve them.[26] We know that healthy motility and properly timed transit of food through the digestive tract supports healthy gut flora and prevents SIBO or the recurrence of it. Having at least three to four hours between meals or practicing intermittent fasting supports the migrating motor complex, which only activates in a fasting state. When the body is allowed a fasting period with no food, the digestive system rests and has more time to repair cells and tissues. However, for some, the stress of IF can overwhelm the body, particularly the thyroid and adrenal glands, so it's best to consult your doctor before trying this strategy.

Parasitic Infections

Parasitic infections of the gut may be more common than you think. You can contract a parasitic infection from pets, drinking contaminated water, or eating contaminated food. Parasites are organisms that must feed off of a host to survive. Depending on the type of parasite, you may have symptoms such as diarrhea, nausea, vomiting, bloating, gas, inability to gain weight, fatigue, muscle cramping, skin rashes, swollen lymph nodes, and stomach cramping that don't go away. Parasites can also live inside the GI tract without you noticing. Some experts say that the most likely cause of chronic diarrhea is due to a parasitic infection.[27] If you think you might be dealing with a parasitic infection, you can get stool and testing with your doctor.

How do you get rid of parasites in your gut? Many natural remedies for eradicating SIBO overlap with treating parasites as well, such as oregano oil, clove oil, and barberry (berberine). [28] As you work to heal your gut, you improve your immune system and the health of your gut microbiome, making it more difficult for parasites to set up camp and survive. Herbal antimicrobial treatments make your body an inhospitable host for parasites, and they die and leave your gut.

Leaky Gut Syndrome

Having a leaky gut means having an increased number of gaps between the cells and junctions in the intestinal lining. In the healthiest state, the gut mucosa, gastrointestinal cells, and gut microbes function together in harmony. This intestinal lining serves as a tight barrier that prevents disease-causing pathogens and harmful toxins from getting inside the body and into the bloodstream, where they can cause us harm. When the cells and junctions are "tight," they help keep what's supposed to stay in the gut inside and what's supposed to stay outside of it out. Imagine gatekeepers at each cell junction, protecting the gut from both sides. This describes the gut lining in an optimal state.

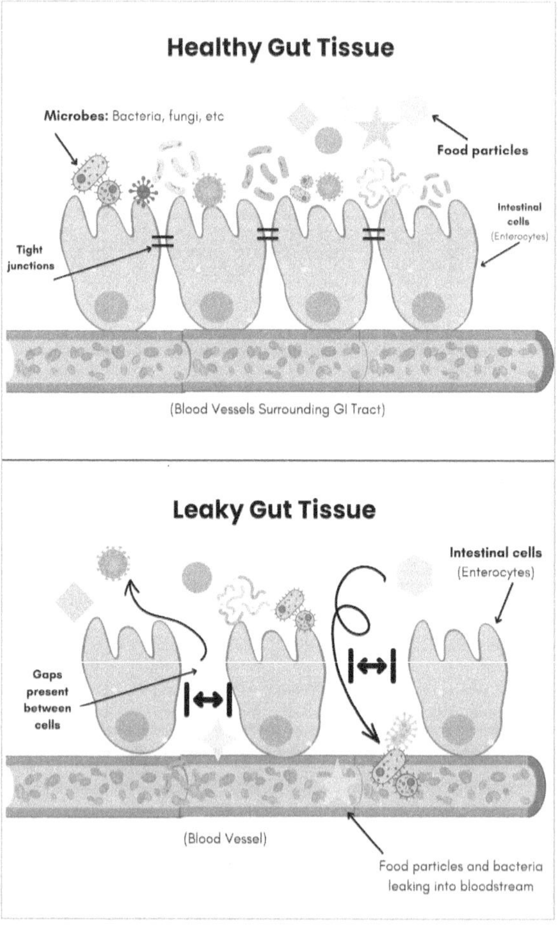

Figure 14

THE INTESTINAL BARRIER is an important part of our small and large intestines. In the previous chapters, we've reviewed how the role of the intestinal wall is to absorb necessary nutrients for our body and prevent the entry of harmful substances or organisms. Inside the gut and intestinal lining are epithelial cells that help extract nutrients from the food we eat and prevent the entry of particles that should stay outside the gut. The healthier your gut, the better this layer of epithelial cells functions as intended, and the junctions between cells remain tight and don't leak.

A layer of mucus lies on top of the epithelial cells, and it operates as another layer of defense for the intestinal cells. Additionally, the mucus layer aids in food passing through the intestines from one end to the other. This mucus layer gets thinner when the gut cells are not healthy and nourished, further lowering defense mechanisms. Additionally, the health of the mucus layer and gut wall also seems to depend on the presence of a certain amount of good bacteria. When the good population decreases, the mucus layer becomes thinner and the tight junctions loosen, resulting in leaky gut.[29]

Our immune system can distinguish between helpful microorganisms in the microbiome and harmful pathogenic ones.[30] Pathogenic refers to the ability to cause disease or infection. The microbiome of healthy individuals has a population of diverse bacteria that aid in providing signals for immune system development and secreting substances that help with processing nutrients from the food we eat. They can even help prevent infections from unhelpful bacteria, viruses, and fungi. Microbial diversity in the gut operates to strengthen and defend you from invaders by supporting digestive tissue health and aiding the immune system.[31] However, when we experience chronic stress from internal and external sources, the gut tissue begins to leak and the intestinal lining and microbiome become disturbed, letting noninvasive bacteria leak out from the inside of the intestines. They get transported to the lymph nodes in the mesenteric region, a layer of tissue that helps hold the intestines in place inside the abdominal cavity. When this happens, it causes an immune response against the microorganisms that would typically not be harmful. This leaking of particles across the barrier activates our immune system, and an inflammatory reaction occurs.

An unhealthy gut is linked with a higher presence of inflammation and intestinal permeability and decreased absorption of B vitamins.[32] Inflammation coincides with many chronic diseases such as arthritis, diabetes, kidney disease, and inflammatory bowel disease. Chronic inflammatory disorders such as these cause more than 50 percent of deaths.[33]

Aren't yet convinced? I don't blame you. Inflammation is microscopic and does damage at a level we can't see right away. A powerful example of how inflammation does harm in secret is Alzheimer's disease. Alzheimer's is a brain condition characterized by nerve cells (called neurons) and brain cells becoming damaged over time. This damage is done faster with inflammation and cytokine activity in the body. Cytokines are proteins that help signal the immune system, similar to how we send text messages back and forth with our friends and family. These messengers signal the immune system to neutralize foreign invaders or fix the damage. It might shock you to learn that Alzheimer's disease begins thirty to fifty years before the first onset of symptoms.[34] Shifting the focus to lowering inflammation by eating better food, balancing your blood sugar, and sleeping more can certainly lower the risk of chronic disease.

Furthermore, when we're internally stressed, corticotrophin-releasing hormone is secreted from the hypothalamus, which signals our pituitary gland to release adrenocorticotropic hormone. Adrenocorticotropic hormone travels through the bloodstream and tells our adrenal glands, which sit on top of our kidneys, to release cortisol into the body.[35] When too much cortisol is circulating, the negative feedback loop turns off the release of corticotropin-releasing hormone. Too much or too little corticotrophin-releasing hormone can provoke anxiety, decrease appetite, and even cause depression, sleep problems, and worsen inflammatory conditions like rheumatoid arthritis, ulcerative colitis, and Crohn's disease.[36]

Higher cortisol levels in the blood signal the body to use more energy resources to deal with stressful situations. It signals our cells and the liver to release glucose into the bloodstream so our body has the energy to deal with the situation. What happens if we have high cortisol levels for a prolonged period? The increased energy demand and the negative feedback loop manifest as blood sugar imbalances, fatigue, chronic stress, bouts of anxiety, and other negative consequences.

Now, you're beginning to see how critical it is to keep external stress levels manageable and uncover any sources of internal stress. We can't avoid the truth—if we want to support the body's gatekeeper and decrease the rate and risk of disease in any area, we should work toward keeping a healthy, balanced gut microbiome.

Why Does Leaky Gut Cause Inflammation?

What is happening deep down at a cellular level when we have a microbial imbalance in our gut? We get more inflammation from the endotoxins released from unhelpful bacteria, such as

LPS. Short for lipopolysaccharide, this compound is found on the surface of gram-negative bacteria such as Escherichia coli (E. Coli), and the overgrowth of it irritates our intestinal lining. LPS can contribute to cellular permeability, which is a term used to describe how leaky a cell's barrier or tissue system is.[37] You can picture high permeability (high leakage) to be similar to a cheap raincoat that lets in more moisture than you would prefer. LPS is not a direct cause of leaky gut, however. It seems that most of the inflammatory signaling that happens with LPS takes place due to the breach in gut wall, allowing gram-negative bacteria to get out into systemic circulation.[38] It's believed the reason someone experiences joint pain with leaky gut is due to endotoxin activity of LPS causing inflammation inside joints. Given that E. coli and other gram-negative bacteria exist in healthy guts all the time, they don't cause issues all on their own. It's more likely that something triggers leaky gut, such eating gluten if you have celiac disease. This results in a protein inside wheat, called gliadin, triggering increases in serum zonulin, a protein responsible for regulating intestinal permeability.[39] [40] [41] This chain reaction causes more intestinal cellular junctions to be unlocked, allowing them to be more permeable. This could also result in gram-negative bacteria escaping into systemic circulation and causing inflammation.

Some inflammation is helpful so the immune system can activate and function as it was designed, but persistent, elevated inflammation damages our body. Every disease begins with inflammation the immune system hasn't diffused. Often, inflammation persists because of what we're eating, toxins, damaged tissues, or a combination of all three. It begins subtly and grows over time. The process has already been in motion by the time you notice changes in your energy, pain, or bloating. But not to worry—with the new information you're learning, you can take simple steps to course correct on your path to a thriving body.

THE LINK BETWEEN GUT DYSBIOSIS, Leaky Gut, and Mental Health

Did you know that the gut and brain communicate through a system called the gut-brain axis (GBA)? The gut and brain communicate back and forth through the vagus nerve in an intricate process influenced by our endocrine (hormone) system, parasympathetic nervous system, and immune system.[42] Hormone function and stress have an undeniable impact on our mental health and digestive health. In research studies, eating disorders, bipolar disorder, depression, inflammatory disease, substance abuse, and bowel disorders often overlap with gut dysbiosis. Even conditions in children such as autism and ADD are linked with increased gut permeability and bacterial imbalances.[43] [44] So, how does this apply to you? For a moment, reflect on your own life over the past few years. Has excessive worrying, anxiety, or depression ever stopped you from taking care of responsibilities, trying new things, or doing things you know you should be doing? If the answer is a resounding yes, consider how positive the impact of increasing your probiotic intake over the next four weeks could be in your life. There's nothing more frustrating than being aware of a desire to have a more positive attitude, feel better, and actually have the kind of life you want while frequently experiencing poor mood and negative emotions that become a regular stumbling block. Thankfully, taking probiotic supplements or probiotic food with the probiotic strain *Lactobacillus* (*L.*) *plantarum* P-8, can support improvement in depression or anxiety.[45] [46] We can't avoid the truth—supporting the gut, the body's gatekeeper, decreases our risk for disease and supports our mental health as well.

<u>KEY TAKEAWAYS:</u>

- Healing your gut from dysbiosis requires restoring the gut wall, maintaining a healthy mucus layer, decreasing harmful bacteria, and diversifying and repopulating the good ones.
- 80 percent or more of IBS cases are misdiagnosed as SIBO.
- To heal your gut, it's important to identify and heal the root cause.
- Herbal antimicrobials help dissolve biofilms around stubborn bad bacteria.
- Leaky gut leads to system-wide, low-grade inflammation.
- Having an unhealthy gut microbiome can increase depression and anxiety.

5

LIFESTYLE FOUNDATIONS FOR SUPPORTING A HEALTHY GUT

While our gut microbiomes have been challenged by our increasingly modern world, you can still decide to change how you live your life, manage stress, and eat to support your gut health.

SUNLIGHT

Some ultraviolet (UV) exposure is healthy because it helps our skin generate vitamin D. Vitamin D and its receptors in the gut support intestinal barrier integrity, meaning that it supports our immune system as well. Aim to get twenty to thirty minutes sun before 10:00 a.m., before UV rays are at their highest, which is between 10:00 a.m. and 4:00 p.m. As we spend more and more time indoors in our modern society life, some of us aren't getting enough vitamin D. Inadequate levels of this vitamin change the microbial population as well and may be contributing to gut dysbiosis.[1] Vitamin D supplementation can be helpful during times when you aren't getting much sunlight, such as winter months in cooler climates. Additionally, allowing sunlight to fall on your face and eyes within ten minutes of waking in the morning will support your gut.

Sleep, Rest, and Circadian Rhythms

Before our modern world, our ancestors operated with circadian rhythms, which is our body's natural clock that helps us wake up in the morning and get tired in the evening. The importance of keeping in sync with your circadian rhythm is to support hormone balance, blood sugar balance, a healthy weight, and gut health.[2] Through research, we've learned that those who experience frequent jet lag and late shift workers have higher blood sugar and higher rates of obesity. Researchers suspect that changes in circadian rhythm also impact gut bacteria in a way that influences blood sugar and weight management. Avoiding caffeine late in the day and getting to sleep between 10:00 p.m. and 12:00 a.m. or around the same time each night supports your body's inner clock.

Tips for Improving Sleep and Circadian Rhythms for Gut and Hormone Balance

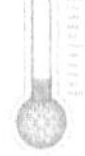

Sleep in a cooler room

Optimal temperature for sleeping is 60-67 degrees F.

Avoid using electronics 2 hours before bed

Blue light from screens blocks melatonin release. Wear blue-light-blocking glasses when using screens before bed.

Block out light

Sleep in a dark room or use black-out curtains to keep light out to minimize waking.

Sound machines

Using a sound machine can help minimize waking if you're easily disturbed by noise.

Avoid caffeine late in the day

Caffeine intake may disrupt ability to feel sleepy at night. Avoid consuming it after 1 p.m.

Maintain a sleep schedule

Try to get to sleep between 10 p.m. to 12 a.m., and around the same time each night.

Figure 15

THE MIGRATING Motor Complex (MMC)

The migrating motor complex (MMC), a propelling motion of the gastrointestinal system, is controlled by the enteric nervous system.[3] It is activated when the body reaches a fasting state, which can be understood as the point when you're finished with your meal and you're "letting it digest." There are four different phases the MMC goes through to support digestion, but it will stop if interrupted by snacking or another meal. A full phase is 130 minutes, so this is when food has been digested and propelled forward into the small bowel. To explain this differently, after food leaves the stomach and enters the small intestine, it gets pushed along the digestive tract while nutrients and water are absorbed until, finally, it is eliminated by the large intestine. To support a healthy microbiome and reduce the risk of SIBO or it's recurrence, avoid snacking between meals and allow three to five hours between eating whenever possible. You wouldn't open up your washing machine in the middle of its rinse cycle just to add more laundry and detergent to it, right? I'm guessing your answer is no—you'd likely let it finish the cycle and start a new load after. Allowing at least three hours between meals for the MMC to complete its cycle before starting to eat again is a similar concept, and it's a good strategy you can use to boost your digestive health and promote healing.

MINERALS

Is the possibility of mineral deficiency on your radar? It certainly didn't occur to me during my twenties. I doubted that supplementing minerals would make any difference at all, until I tried them and stopped feeling so anxious, depressed, and tired all day long. Just like me in my twenties, many Americans don't get enough minerals in their diet. Disorders involving the digestive system and inflammatory bowel disease elevate risk for multiple mineral deficiencies because they aren't properly absorbed from the food you eat.[4] Not eating a wide variety of whole foods and consuming a diet high in saturated fats and processed foods stripped of their nutrients leaves 50 percent of Americans deficient in magnesium and other essential nutrients.[5] Magnesium plays an important role in gut health because it supports muscle relaxation and helps regulate inflammation, which we want to keep low. If you've been diagnosed with high blood pressure, heart disease, or kidney disease, it's likely your doctor or nutritionist has told you that you need to cut back on salt because it can cause you to retain water and increases blood pressure. Refined sea salt, regular table salt, has had its trace minerals stripped away and often has anti-caking and other additives inside, leaving it void of the health benefits it once had. Additives and chemicals like this can contribute to leaky gut. What you want to do instead is look for Himalayan sea salt, which has an estimated sixty to eighty trace minerals in it, like potassium, calcium, and magnesium. Adding a little bit of Himalayan sea salt to your food is a better choice for health, as it can be another way to get your daily minerals.

Food Eating Techniques

Did you know that chewing your food twenty to thirty times before swallowing can reduce bloating and acid reflux? Chewing food adequately allows the enzymes in your saliva to begin breaking food down and can support digestive health. Additionally, a short walk after eating keeps blood sugar levels stable and may improve weight loss.[6] While walking, gravity is working to your advantage as food exits the stomach and heads into the small intestine, reducing the chance of trapped air resulting in gas as digestion continues.

PHYSICAL ACTIVITY

Low-intensity exercise such as walking and strength training can actually reduce the time that stool is in the colon, which is a protective measure for SIBO and keeping a healthy mucus layer. This shows positive effects of the colon being protected from cancer and inflammatory bowel disease.[7] Contrastingly, exercise at higher frequency and intensity can actually increase gut leakiness and inflammation.[8] Timing your physical activities to be around thirty minutes after eating a meal not only supports digestion, it is also a way to prevent blood sugar from spiking too high, protecting you from damage that persistently high blood sugar causes over years.[9]

It's important to do movement that you enjoy, such as dancing, sports, or hiking. Adding things you like to do that often overlap with social time is a more sustainable way to keep physical activity enjoyable for the long-term. Focus less on repetitive, forced exercise for the sake of "getting it out of the way," as this will take away from a feeling of balance and enjoyment in life. We'll go over how to balance gut health, physical activity, and weight loss effectively without tanking your metabolism and hormones in chapter 11.

Stress Reduction

As you can imagine, physical and mental stress and the influence they have on the body can be an infinite loop. Lifestyle choices, stress, the gut, and our systems inside of us are in a bio-feedback loop, continuously communicating. Depression and stress promote expansion of unhelpful gut bacteria and leaky gut, and vice versa.[10] With dysbiosis, neurotransmitters that the gut controls are dysregulated, leading to chronic inflammation and leaky gut. If you continue doing the same actions, you'll stay on the same loop. So, interrupt it with stress-reduction measures, probiotics, and healthy choices, and you'll be changing the communication in a positive way. Taking time out to engage in prayer, mindfulness, breathing, and meditative practices supports expansion of healthy gut microbes and decreases inflammation as a result.[11]

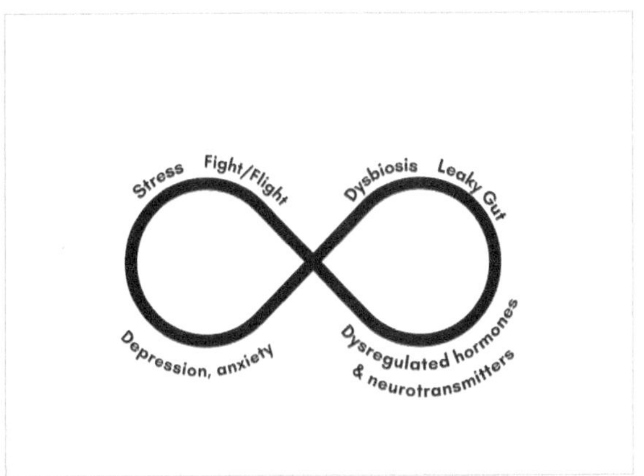

Figure 16

Controlling your breathing through a method known as diaphragmatic breathing (DB) sends calming signals through the phrenic and vagus nerves and calms the nervous system. From there, stress responses are decreased, which supports digestion as well as heart health, the immune system, and mental health. It can even increase antioxidants and stress from exercise for athletes.[12]

Diaphragmatic Breathing in 3 Steps

1

Lying down, place one hand on your chest and one on your stomach. This is to help you understand what an expanding diaphragm feels like.

2

Begin by inhaling for 6 seconds, and letting a controlled exhale out over 6 seconds. Breathe in deeply, allowing your stomach to expand beneath your hand.

3

Repeat this breath cycle for at least 5 minutes and find yourself feeling more deeply relaxed. It may take several tries to learn how to properly expand your diaphragm.

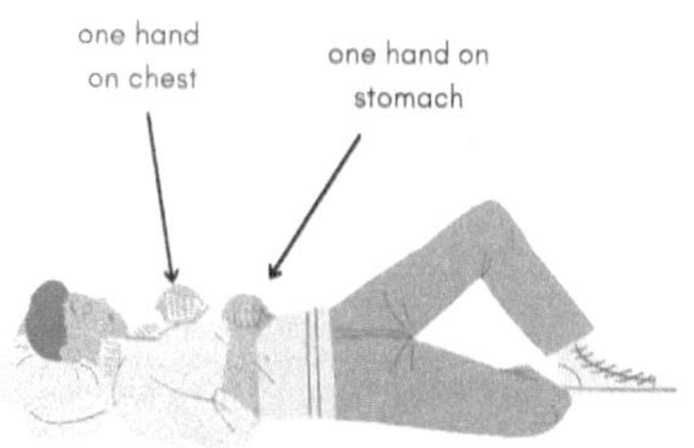

Figure 17

ENJOY YOUR LIFE

I'll take the opportunity to bring up a topic you may not have expected to be in this book: having fun. Lately, joy and play has received more attention as conversations about mental health are stirring post-pandemic. During the worldwide shutdown, many of us noticed that our lives froze, suspended for an indefinite amount of time. Collectively, our anxiety skyrocketed, and many of us noticed how much our mental health needed rescuing.

Have you ever felt your mind begin to race when you're going out with a friend for a dinner and a glass of wine, thinking to yourself how you're going to fit an extra workout in to burn off the calories you consumed that evening? I'll be honest, I used to do this, but I stopped after learning about how impactful enjoying the present moment with someone I care about is, as it actually has stress-decreasing effects. Perhaps it would be better to allow a balance and become more relaxed about getting food and exercise done perfectly. Many people are unaware that loneliness causes the same amount of risk as smoking does for heart attacks.[13] Can you imagine how intentional people would take their relationships, community, and social life if they knew? (Well now you know, and you can share the news.) Perhaps the education system would begin teaching us more about creating and maintaining positive relationships for a lifetime while we're in school. Negative emotions and stress that comes about because of how we feel on a regular basis affect the inside of us and, most importantly, the heart. Why are the centenarians in Italy enjoying wine, eating pasta and full-fat cheese, and living beyond one hundred years, all while maintaining their health? Don't drinking and eating these kinds of foods increase the risk of heart disease? It's because they're consistently surrounding themselves with the people who matter most to them and enjoying these moments.

The fact of the matter is keeping enjoyable company with others where you're sharing belly laughs and experiences and making memories creates an inner response that can reduce stress and add years to your life. These one-hundred-year-olds reveal again and again that food isn't the sole influencing factor on your longevity and quality of health.

KEY TAKEAWAYS:

- Your lifestyle and stress levels influence the health of your gut.
- Diaphragmatic breathing and sleeping adequately are helpful stress-reduction strategies for healing your gut.
- Lack of community, isolation, and loneliness are perhaps some of the biggest stressors on your mind and body.

6

____

FOOD MISCONCEPTIONS: HAVE WE BEEN MISLED ABOUT HEALTHY EATING ALL ALONG?

Imagine the composition of your body in cells. Our microscopic cells make up 10 percent of what's living in our physical body, and the other 90 percent are microorganisms living in our gut, skin, and other tissues.[1] The food we eat has a profound impact on our gut microbiota. As we've discussed earlier, the food we eat has the power to either cause our intestinal barrier and gut microbiota to be fortified and resilient or tear them down little by little. The link between the gut microbiome and common chronic diseases such as diabetes, heart disease, and Parkinson's disease continues to be revealed through research, so it is imperative that we learn how to take care of our gut and then do so.[2] The world has more knowledge about food and its interaction with the human body than ever before, so why are we still so confused about the nutrition our bodies need for nourishment and balance? Many of us have been told to eliminate dairy and gluten (and perhaps other foods) with no explanation detailing why, so we just think they're bad for us and never move past surface-level understanding. Here are three possible reasons we're confused about what to eat to be healthy:

1. Food companies market their products without consideration of the impact on health.
2. Numerous experts and gurus promote particular food ideologies and diets as "the one" for all people, without enough emphasis on the bio-individuality of people. What is good for one person is another person's poison.
3. We are mostly unaware of the basics of nutrition and that consumption of whole food nutrition is the foundation for a healthy body and longevity.

FOOD MARKETING

Food marketing influences us, and the way it's done often causes us to believe things that aren't necessarily true about food and its relation to our general health. Since the 1950s, processing food has helped the economy become more profitable, but unfortunately, it does not provide the same benefits for our health.[3] The media then writes a headline that profoundly impacts our understanding of the benefit and manipulates us into believing that eating that food will lower our risk for heart disease. As an example, the macadamia nut company Royal Hawaiian Nuts petitioned the FDA to be able to use this statement on their food packaging: "supportive but nonconclusive evidence states eating 1.5 oz of macadamia nuts daily as part of a diet low in saturated fat and cholesterol and not resulting in increased intake of saturated fat or calories may reduce the risk of coronary heart disease."[4] In 2017, the FDA made a statement in response to this, along with a movement to require more disclaimers on the packaging. They wanted to avoid being held responsible if someone felt the health information they read on these packages was misleading. On top of the selective information advertised, the companies making the products fund research to find health benefits to consuming these foods. The petition Royal Hawaiian Macadamia Nuts brought to the FDA included a research study funded by Hershey's, a seller of chocolate-covered macadamia nuts. Sellers marketing their food know that a health statement from the FDA has the power to push their message effectively to the masses and that people will trust it.

Being well and preventing disease is less about whether you choose to eat a particular food for the health benefit it provides and more about all the food you're eating collectively. The point is that it's not one food that will help lower your risk of heart disease and cancer; it's all the food you're eating, your lifestyle, environment, and genetics, in an amalgamation that influences your health outcomes.

THE WIDE VARIETY of Expert Recommendations

Why are there so many experts recommending completely different diets? This will stump you until you understand how bio-individuality and personalized nutrition can make or break someone's health. It's not that there is only one truth and multiple experts are wrong. One of the keys to healing your gut and optimizing your wellness is acknowledging the philosophy of bio-individuality, which states that each person has unique needs. It supports the idea that although a particular food or diet may be suitable for one individual, it can inflame the next person.[5] So while one person may benefit from a plant-based diet, another person might benefit from a ketogenic diet instead. How can this be when those diets are drastically different? This is the wonder of bio-individuality at work.

. . .

Whole Food Nutrition

In addition to the never-ending dietary theories we have to sort through, more uncertainty develops when we remember that what was recommended as a balanced diet thirty years ago is much different today. In 1992, the United States government published the Food Pyramid Guide to show Americans what was healthy to eat. With the rates of obesity, diabetes, heart disease, hormone imbalances, digestive disorders, and insulin resistance today, we know the recommendation in 1992 to have most of our food intake come from bread, pasta, and grains wasn't right.

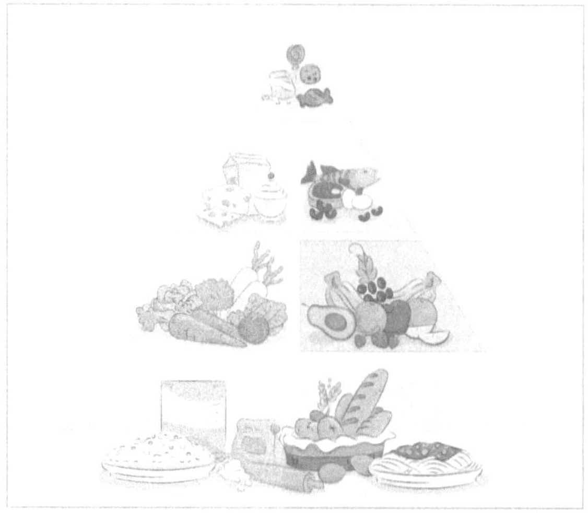

Figure 18 - The Food Pyramid 1992

AFTER 2005, the pyramid got flipped on its side. The recommendations were updated to vertical slivers in the shape of a triangle, with the advice being to eat mostly grains, pasta, and bread, and eat the smallest amount of fat possible. Still, our disease rates and waist circumferences continued to increase. We weren't getting better, we were getting worse! In 2011, the pyramid was scrapped, and the round plate entered. The USDA MyPlate includes grains, vegetables, fruits, protein, and dairy sections. The MyPlate is the most balanced plate yet, but a few things were left out. There is no reference to water, and again, no fat intake, which leaves us guessing what and how much to drink. And where are the nuts and olive oil? After looking at this plate, you might wonder if you should be eating them. If you're confused, you're not alone.

In 2016, the World Health Organization made a statement that knocked us out of our seats: nearly 40 percent of the world's population was overweight, and 25 percent of that number was considered obese. Worldwide obesity has tripled since 1975, and in 2020, 39 million children under the age of five were overweight.[6] What caused this increase? We've been told what's healthy for the last thirty years. Shouldn't following the guidelines given to us by people in charge of looking after the public's health make us healthy instead of sicker? Following the dietary history of the last half century reveals the answers.

In the 1970s, the federal government established the Senate Select Committee on Nutrition and Human Needs to intersect the agriculture and food production industries with the welfare of people. This was when guidelines around food began to emerge from the government, and one of the critical points targeted was lowering dietary fat intake. In the 1940s, coronary heart disease was the leading cause of death. As a result, many studies were conducted to unearth the cause of increased risk for heart disease. Since some studies suggested a diet high in saturated fats and cholesterol was causing this increase, the low-fat diet became the gold standard for improving heart health, even though some of the studies could not deliver supporting evidence. Many experts argued for the low-fat diet approach using this point as support.

By the 1980s, the federal government recommended a low-fat diet for everyone, regardless of their heart health or weight status. A low-fat diet was considered to be 30 percent or less of daily calories coming from dietary fat sources. At first, the food industry was not happy about the new recommendations. There were unreconciled questions from the studies that had failed to bring evidence supporting low-fat as the best way to eat. But then it dawned on companies that this was an incredible opportunity to make a profit. Food manufacturing companies began to create low-fat products and market them to Americans. What's concerning is that these companies had to increase the number of refined carbohydrates in low-fat products to keep the flavor and texture, which was later connected to metabolic diseases such as diabetes and an increase in triglycerides. Research unveils that diets high in refined carbohydrates and low in unsaturated fat can lower HDL and decrease heart protection in the body.[7] The government said to remove the fat to reduce heart disease, but we didn't know we'd be paying for it with increasing weight and diabetes.

Once the doctors and federal government label a diet as the best for weight loss and heart protection, it grows legs and takes on a life of its own. By the 1980s and 1990s, the low-fat diet had caught fire, and consumers wanted more low-fat products to add to their pantry. Due to the demand, food manufacturing companies began pumping out more products labeled as "low fat" that ironically contained just as many calories as the higher-fat products but were filled with more refined sugars and carbohydrates to maintain flavor quality. Despite that fact, the production and marketing continued. What do you do as a business in a world of economic shifts and trends? You adapt to them, or you face the likely possibility of going out of business. After much arguing and debate, the food pyramid was born in 1992 in the United States, and we were stuck with the government's stamp of approval and the mass message for the next thirteen years: low-fat is best, and most of our food should come from refined carbohydrate sources such as bread, pasta, and rice. What took this movement even further was that the American Heart Association (AHA) began a program in 1988 to parallel the low-fat diet recommendations, where they would allow food companies to pay to have a "heart-healthy" label printed on their packaging. The AHA could endorse food if it met its low saturated fat and cholesterol standards. Forget about the refined carbohydrates and sugar inside each of these products. If it was low in fat and cholesterol, it was considered healthy. The program was withdrawn in 1990, after people argued a fair point: fresh produce isn't labeled and therefore could not get the AHA's approval label. The issue was if people were magnetized to food labeled with the AHA's standards for a heart-healthy diet, they could be left thinking packaged and processed foods were the healthiest, possibly decreasing their purchase and consumption of fresh foods. The program was reopened in 1993, and in the next five years, six hundred products were certified as heart-healthy, including foods such as Kellogg's cereal and Pop-Tarts.[8] What's wrong about this is that a sleeve of Pop-Tarts has just as much sugar as a serving of Ben and Jerry's ice cream.

How did the obesity rates of the entire world triple since the low-fat recommendations have been widely accepted and followed? It's complicated. In developing countries, many struggling with high rates of obesity have foods available that are processed and high in fats, sugars, and salt and lack proper nutrients. The focus on nutrition in other countries has been influenced by the economy and what was low in cost. In developing countries with these types of foods available, it's not uncommon to observe malnutrition and obesity increasing simultaneously due to the high sugar content yet lack of nutrients in the food.[9]

Then we have the obesity rates rising in highly developed countries. Low-fat foods have added sugars and refined carbohydrates to make up for the taste and texture when fats are removed. Removing fat decreases the satiation value of foods, causing you to want to eat more to trigger the fullness hormone from your brain. High sugar and refined carbohydrates lack richness in their nutrient profile, which further subtracts from satiation and our body's needs. High consumption of foods containing refined carbs and sugars spike blood sugar, invoking a high insulin response and leading to metabolic issues such as type 2 diabetes. Even more problems arise from eating a diet low in unsaturated fats and refined carbohydrates. This contributes to elevated triglycerides and low high-density lipoprotein (HDL) in many people. This leads to higher levels of low-density lipoprotein (LDL), which is more likely to cause atherosclerotic plaques in the vessels around the body and our heart, increasing the risk of having a blockage and leading to a heart attack.[10] HDL is heart-protective, and low levels can cause a problem. High levels of LDL, low levels of HDL, high blood sugar levels, and insulin resistance create an inflammatory and deadly recipe for health problems such as strokes, myocardial infarctions (heart attacks), vision problems, heart disease, and circulation issues that compromise blood flow to limbs and fingers.

The real goal behind becoming healthy is to have an appropriate cholesterol ratio and stable blood glucose management without insulin resistance. Accomplish these things, and you reduce your risk for nearly every disease. Weight loss, brain health, sleep, and internal stress improve, which helps you feel better, look better, and live longer.

<u>KEY TAKEAWAYS:</u>

- The government's recommendations over the past 50 years to eat less dietary fat as an effort to decrease heart disease has come with increased rates of diabetes and obesity.
- The right kind of dietary fat is essential for maintaining healthy HDL cholesterol levels.
- LDL cholesterol ("bad" cholesterol) does not cause heart disease independently. Blockages in the arteries around the heart and throughout the body occur when there are high levels of LDL cholesterol accompanied by high levels of blood sugar and inflammation.

7

UNDERSTANDING HOW TO EAT FOR A HEALTHY GUT

What role does gut health play in metabolic health and heart disease? Metabolic syndrome and gut dysbiosis are often found together, manifesting as low inflammation levels that destroy the gut wall. Byproducts of the damage and inflammation create insulin resistance and can push metabolic syndrome further along, becoming a vicious cycle of poor gut and metabolic health.[1]

Metabolic health is another way to describe the status of our metabolism. Metabolism refers to your body's ability to properly respond to the food you're eating and use it in a good way.[2] Our metabolism, hormones, and gut health are inseparable and are woven together intricately. If their dance is disrupted by stress in one area, the other areas suffer, and homeostasis, our body's balancing system, must restabilize everything.

Multiple factors can influence our metabolism and the body's response to certain foods—chronic dieting coupled with prolonged periods of high-intensity physical activity, food sensitivities, and chronic stress, to name a few. But one thing is for sure, and that is how and what we're regularly eating is a large deciding factor in how healthy our metabolism is. Every single day, we make choices that will impact the health of our body, months and years from now. This is actually really good news, because it means we are completely in control when improving metabolic health. Have you ever known someone who claims that just looking at a donut makes them put on five pounds? We're intelligent enough to know that this is not how the body truly works; however, the statement is relatable for some and may actually reflect that the person doesn't have a great metabolism. To look at it from another angle, if their metabolic health got the support it needed through upgraded food and lifestyle decisions, a few months later, this same person might report that they ate two donuts from the breakroom on Friday, but they were pleasantly surprised that they hadn't gained any pounds when they weighed in on Monday.

Gradually stacking up small, health-minded decisions with food over time can mean the difference between a getting slapped with a fancy new diagnosis of autoimmune disease or diabetes not too far down the road or receiving a clean bill of health from your doctor way past your 40's and 50's. Our wonderful bodies are so intelligent and will always instinctually work toward healing any imbalance. We simply have to remove what bothers it and in exchange provide what will help it heal. You hold the future in your own hands with this one!

WE'VE KNOWN for over twenty years that insulin resistance and poor metabolic health is scarily correlated with plaque formations, poor cholesterol, and heart health.[3] What we desperately need is to follow up on this knowledge with questions about how to make choices with food to reverse these problems and restore what's been damaged.

But how do you leverage nutrition to help repair metabolic problems and gut health? This chapter will allow you to further develop your understanding of how to use nutrition to your advantage while finding a balance between all foods.

MACRONUTRIENTS

Carbohydrates, protein, and fat make up macronutrients, and these are energy-supplying components that come from what we eat. Let's take a look at each one.

Carbohydrates

Carbohydrates take a lead role as the body's preferred fuel source. They provide the body with sustained energy, can assist with preserving muscle mass, and fuel our brains. Carbohydrates come in different forms, including starches, sugars, and fiber. Starchy carbohydrates are grains, fruits, bread, pasta, and vegetables like potatoes and corn.[4] Sugar is found in a delightful array such as inside dates, cane sugar, and honey. Fiber is mainly found in plant-based foods like grains, vegetables, legumes, nuts, and seeds.

Carbohydrates can come in refined form (aka processed) and unrefined (known as whole and unprocessed). During the processing of carbs, such as white rice or refined wheat, they become stripped of their bran and germ, which contain many nutrients, so their original health benefits are drastically reduced. Refined carbohydrates are broken down by enzymes and quickly digested, which causes a spike and then a drop in blood sugar levels. This dramatic fluctuation in blood sugar can feel like a quick burst of energy followed by a crash in a couple of hours. This also may increase cravings and feelings of hunger soon after eating. I'm not sure about you, but I prefer to start my day with a high energy level that remains stable. Hold onto this thought because, in a moment, we'll cover a few of my favorite ways to eat for an energetic morning.

Additionally, carbs are simple or complex. Simple carbohydrates can come in whole food form, like fruit, and processed, like cane sugar. Simple carbs are composed of sugars that are one or two chains long and are easier to break down for energy.

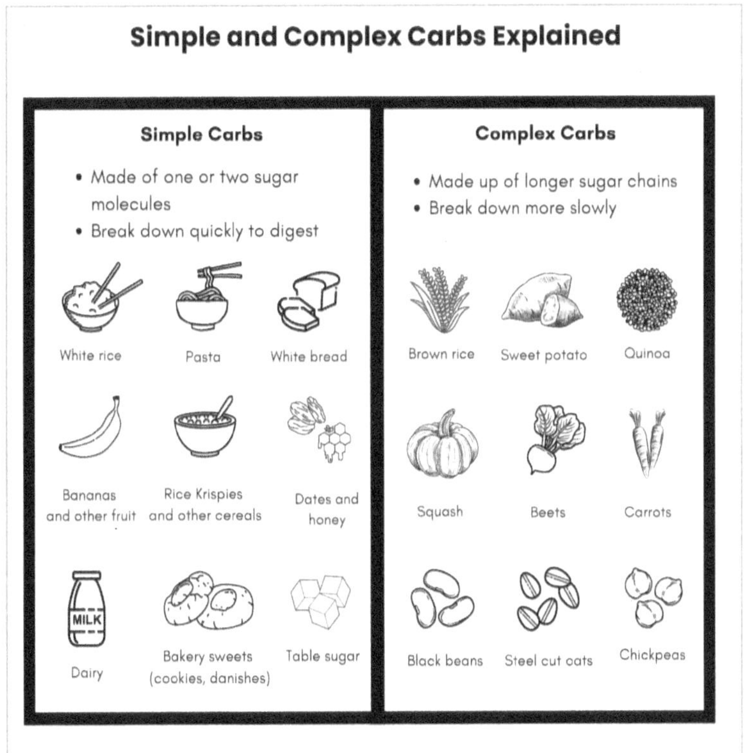

Figure 19

YOU MAY WONDER if simple carbs from whole foods are okay to eat due to their effect on blood sugar. When deciding which foods to eat, remember that whole foods have their original macronutrient profile intact, which is what's important. The fiber, vitamins, minerals, macronutrients, and water are all still there and are essential for each system in your body to thrive. A simple carbohydrate, such as an orange or a white potato, can still be a good choice for gut health and overall wellness because it also contains other helpful nutrients and fiber. Oranges don't need to be fortified with any vitamins. Whole foods are not processed and stripped of nutrients like a bowl of Cocoa Puffs. With this in mind, however, it's essential to recall what your goals are for your health and make food decisions based on a balance between that and what you genuinely enjoy eating. There is a way to reach your goals without cutting out foods or food groups altogether; we'll review this in a moment.

Fiber

A secret weapon of choice for gut health, dietary fiber can help feed the gut microbes, balance hormones, reduce insulin resistance, and aid in weight loss. Classification of fiber can become confusing, but the vital thing to remember is that fiber is considered either soluble or insoluble. Both varieties aid in digestion differently. Soluble fibers dissolve in water. They are also easily digested by the gut bacteria to create energy byproducts called short-chain fatty acids (SCFAs). SCFAs help heal insulin resistance and keep the intestinal wall and mucus strengthened, which explains why keeping a healthy gut can be a helpful ally to our metabolic health as well.[5] Examples of soluble fibers are inulin, pectin, beta-glucans, fructooligosaccharides (found in fruits, vegetables and legumes), and galactooligosaccharides (found in dairy products, some beans, and root vegetables). Insoluble fiber doesn't ferment as quickly by gut bacteria and helps draw water into the colon, adding bulk to stool for the body to pass it more easily. Insoluble (indigestible) fibers are cellulose, lignin, and hemicellulose, which can be consumed by eating grains and seeds.

Prebiotic foods have fibers that cannot be digested. They feed our gut microbes and help them to provide energy to us. You can take a ton of probiotics and repopulate the good bacteria, but if you're not feeding them with prebiotic fibers, they won't stick around very long. All plant foods and some animal-based foods have prebiotics in them, but the foods listed below have the highest content of these fibers.

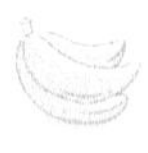
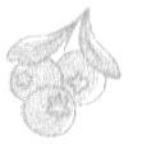
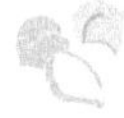

Prebiotic Foods List

- Bananas
- Jerusalem artichoke
- Pears
- Chicory root
- Lemons
- Papaya
- Garlic
- Onions
- Shallots
- Green onions
- Leeks
- Cabbage
- Chickpeas
- Lentils
- Beans
- Apples
- Watermelon
- Grapefruit
- Acacia powder
- Allulose
- Bran
- Blackberries
- Barley
- Oats
- Almonds
- Pistachios
- Flaxseeds

Figure 20

<u>SUGAR</u>

Sugar has been demonized for being addictive. Have you ever experienced fiend-like cravings for sugar? It's like a strong urge to eat something that tastes sweet, and you feel out of control around food, which leads to overeating or binge-eating. After the temporary high is over, many find themselves overweight, tired, and feeling puffy, bloated, and dehydrated. There is a neurobiological reason you can't kick sugar cravings no matter what you try, which debunks the idea you should just use self-control. Self-control and discipline have their appropriate place, but this only goes so far when your body produces a neurochemical response. When we eat sugar, our brain releases opioids and dopamine, a neurotransmitter from the basal ganglia. Dopamine is part of the pleasure and reward center, and combined with the opioid release, the brain becomes conditioned to the release of these chemicals when sugar is consumed, and the neurological circuits in our brains adapt. If continued, whether it's sugar or a drug, a tolerance develops as the receptors become less sensitive to the neurochemicals.[6] This makes you require more to induce the same feeling of pleasure. When a person is healthy, exercising self-control over their impulses is easier because there is balance in the prefrontal cortex in the circuits that help with decision-making and judgment. When the brain's circuits are altered with addiction, self-control is decreased. This response is not exclusive to sugar or addictive drugs and can also happen with artificial and nonglycemic sweeteners, as it is related to the "addictive" portion of the sweet flavor, not the sugar itself. When taken away, the body goes through a withdrawal process that can be pretty unpleasant, with chills, shakiness, anxiety, and headaches.

Refined sugar consumption can negatively affect the gut by modulating the population of microbes. Eating more refined sugars encourages candida, a naturally occurring fungus, and other microbes to multiply, which can grow out of healthy proportion. If your immune system is compromised, you will be at a higher risk for more infections. Yeast infections, infections of the blood, and oral thrush can result if you have an overgrowth of candida. Therefore, reducing refined sugar and high-lactose dairy products can assist in managing candida overgrowth and dysbiosis in the gut.[7] If you have SIBO, swapping out sugar, milk, and processed cheeses (such as Velveeta or Kraft) becomes especially important and will influence your ability to rebalance your gut microbes.

BEFORE YOU GET DISCOURAGED and ask if you need to cut out sugar completely, let's bring up something important. Additional reasons for sugar or carbohydrate cravings are stress, lack of sleep, dehydration, and cutting out foods or food groups altogether. The critical piece here is that cravings signal an imbalance of something. The lack of balance could come from chronically sleeping four to five hours per night, which would not allow your brain or body adequate resources to function and therefore cause cravings. If continued, the lack of sleep will increase stress on the adrenal glands and increase circulating cortisol, and there is more to heal.

Here is where the discussion about sugar versus nonglycemic sweeteners gets more interesting. Sugar can negatively influence the gut microbiome in ways natural, nonglycemic sweeteners do not. Sugar reduces diversity in the gut, causing the population of proteobacteria to increase and the amount of bacteroidetes to decrease.[8] Additionally, the candida population may grow. This shift is connected with metabolic disorders such as diabetes and inflammatory bowel diseases. Therefore, by manipulating the gut bacteria, eating a high amount of sugar in foods can cause an increase in inflammation of the gut. This inflammation increases gut leakiness or permeability and is associated with more fat accumulation and a fatty liver.

When sugar is eaten, converted to glucose, and absorbed through the stomach, it goes into your bloodstream and circulates the body, invoking an insulin response to bring the sugar to the organs and tissues than need it. Whatever is left over after the liver is done processing gets stored as glycogen in muscle tissue and then converted to fat for storage once glycogen stores are full. This is where a nonglycemic sweetener can help out as you're looking to balance your gut microbiome and blood sugar. The best nonglycemic, natural sweeteners are monk fruit extract, allulose, and stevia. Additionally, if one of your desires is to reduce body fat around your waist or in general, nonglycemic sweeteners are a great way to continue eating foods you enjoy and successfully reach your goal without falling into a toxic relationship with sweet foods.

Monk fruit extract comes from the monk fruit plant in Asia, is 100 percent natural, and the taste closely resembles sugar. It may also help with digestion. Allulose is a sweetener that can be harvested from figs, raisins, or corn. It's about 70 percent as sweet as regular sugar and has a gentle, sugar-like taste. Stevia is extracted from the leaves of the stevia plant and is one hundred to three hundred times as sweet as regular sugar. Stevioside, purified stevia, is the only form approved by the FDA, as whole-leaf stevia has been found to cause kidney damage. Some say stevia tastes bitter and don't prefer to use it as a sweetener. Liquid stevia is my favorite form to use when baking or mixing smoothies to add a little more sweetness, and it comes in mint and chocolate flavors.

The Smart Way to Eat Carbs

Are you confused about how carbs affect your body? Some people find the need to cut out all carbs and sweet-flavored foods to meet their health goals, but there is a more balanced approach. For most people, cutting out foods or entire food groups for life is usually not sustainable. It's common to see opposing information and advice for the consumption of carbohydrates during a scroll session on your favorite social media platform. Descriptive words like complex, simple, processed, unprocessed, and whole can complicate your understanding of how to eat carbs. How can you sort through all this information and make the best decision for your body? Consider the example of eating a bowl of Cocoa Puffs for breakfast versus a bowl of steel-cut oatmeal. The cereal is made of refined rice or corn flour and corn syrup, which will be broken down and digested quickly compared to steel-cut oats. One way to understand how a carbohydrate might break down in the body is to look at its glycemic index (GI), which is based on how quickly the carb raises your blood sugar after eating.[9] Cocoa Puffs cereal has a GI of seventy-seven,[10] which is considered high. Steel-cut oats have a glycemic index of forty-two, which will provide a slower release of glucose into the bloodstream.

Additionally, protein and fat macronutrients in food also influence the release of glucose into the bloodstream. Steel-cut oats have fourteen grams of protein per half cup uncooked, and the protein delays carbohydrate breakdown even more because the stomach is busy breaking down protein into amino acids. Add some nut butter to your oatmeal and a handful of berries. Now you have fat, slow-burning carbs, protein, and antioxidants in your meal, further adding to the satiation value and providing more energy. Not only do steel-cut oats offer diversity in nutrient profile, but the timed-release breakdown of nutrients also delivers stable energy for hours. You won't be scrounging around for a quick snack two hours after breakfast.

<u>Glycemic Index of Foods</u>[11]

Low (<55)	Medium (56-69)	High (70+)
• 1 apple	• ¾ cup cooked brown rice	• 1 white potato
• 1 orange	• Three rice cakes	• French fries
• ½ cup kidney beans	• 1 slice of whole-grain bread	• Refined breakfast cereal (Cocoa Puffs)
• ½ cup black beans	• ¼ cup whole grain pasta, cooked	• 12 oz can of soda
• ½ cup lentils	• 1 sweet potato	• Candy bars (KitKat, Snickers, Reese's cups)
• ¼ cup cashews	• 1 banana	• 12 oz fruit juice (fresh and store-bought)
• ¼ cup peanuts	• One slice of rye bread	• 1 cup white rice
• 1 cup cooked carrots		• 1 cup white flour pasta
• 1 cup unsweetened almond milk		• 1 cup oat milk
• ¾ cup cooked steel-cut oats		

Table 1

Making smart decisions around carbohydrates becomes critical when dealing with binge-eating habits. While a large part of binge-eating is emotional, there are also physical contributing factors. Hormones in our brain signal cravings and increased appetite if we're not feeding our body with enough macronutrients and micronutrients to meet our daily needs. Whether intentional or not, nutrient and calorie restriction coupled with skipping breakfast or having too many hours between meals is a setup for binge-eating. Restriction of carbs and sugar is also not a long-term answer to issues with cravings and binges. If you eliminate carbs and sugar for that reason, you're not finding out the reason you're experiencing cravings in the first place.

PROTEINS

When digested, each gram of protein breaks down into a diverse array of amino acids. Each type of protein has a slightly different amino acid profile and can help support the body's processes. Protein is essential for muscle growth, maintenance, and for integrity of the gut lining. Interestingly, the amino acids glutamine and glycine can help reverse any damage to the gut from diseases[12] and help repair the integrity of the gut afterward. Glutamine also plays a critical role in helping the body produce the antioxidant glutathione, which allows the immune system to neutralize foreign invaders. You can also supplement glutamine. Along with many others, I have had noticeable reduction in bloating and digestive symptoms after mixing two to three grams of L-glutamine powder in my water throughout the day. As you're improving the diversity of your diet to heal your gut, practice bringing in one or two foods rich in glutamine and glycine every week until you have rotated through the whole list. See Table 2 for a list of foods high in these amino acids. You'll notice that the suggested meals and recipes in the Four Week Gut Health Reset Plan have a variety of foods that include glutamine and glycine.

GLUTAMINE AND GLYCINE-RICH <u>Foods</u>[13]

Glutamine-Rich Foods	Glycine-Rich Foods
• Seafood	• Grass-fed steak
• Grass-fed kefir and ricotta cheese	• Grass-fed ground beef
• Grass-fed, free-range meat (chicken, beef, lamb)	• Turkey
• Red cabbage	• Chicken
• Eggs	• Pork
• Yogurt	• Peanuts
• Soybeans	• Salmon
• Kidney beans	• Quinoa
• Parsley	• Hard cheese (i.e., parmesan)
• Dark leafy greens (kale, spinach, cilantro, lettuce, radish greens)	• Soybeans
• Grass-fed and finished organ meat (liver, heart, testicle, ovaries, kidney, thymus, tripe)	• Almonds
• Chickpeas	• Eggs
• Lentils	• Beans

Table 2

HOW MUCH PROTEIN should we be eating? There have been claims that a diet high in protein (getting 30 to 50 percent of daily calories from protein) puts stress on the kidneys and heart, but studies have revealed that eating more protein does not increase the risk of diseases in these organs.[14] Other evidence shows that a high-protein diet without adequate dietary fiber can cause a shift in the gut microbiota that allows for a decrease in tight junction proteins and increased inflammation. With the presence of inflammation, the impairment in the intestine's ability to defend against foreign pathogens increases leakiness in the gut lining.[15] Along with this change comes an increased risk for obesity and type 2 diabetes. When choosing protein intake for a healthy gut, the amount of dietary fiber you eat makes a noticeable difference. Maintaining a fiber intake of around twenty to thirty-five grams per day will help feed your gut bacteria and help produce an adequate amount of short-chain fatty acids that the neurological and immune systems can use to thrive. For the standard adult who is mostly sedentary, keep your protein intake at no less than 0.8g/kg of your body weight. For example, if you weigh one hundred sixty-five pounds (seventy-five kg), to prevent your body from breaking down muscle tissue so it can meet your daily amino acid requirements, your protein intake should not fall below sixty grams daily. If you have an active job or exercise several times per week for at least thirty minutes, your protein requirements will increase, and you will need a range of 0.9-1.2g more per kg of body weight to provide adequate amino acids and prevent muscle breakdown. So, it's most beneficial to eat a moderate protein intake balanced with enough fiber for healthy gut maintenance. Aim to get 20 to 30 percent of your daily calories from protein. A quick rule of thumb is to eat twenty to thirty grams of protein and seven to twelve grams of dietary fiber at each meal. Consuming 20g of collagen peptides from marine animals or grass-fed cattle can add a strong leg to your gut healing plan because it has been shown to reduce bloating and digestive symptoms.[16] Collagen is a protein found in skin, ligaments, cartilage, bone, and connective tissues. Sources of food high in collagen are grass-fed beef and organ meats, bone broth, and collagen supplements.

Protein diversity makes a difference as well. Eating a variety of proteins from animal and plant sources presents the body with a diverse supply of amino acids. To illustrate this, instead of eating only eggs, chicken breast, and white fish as protein sources, diversify your choices. Rotate in beans, wild salmon, grass-fed beef, soy protein, chicken thighs, grass-fed beef organs, bone broth, collagen, elk, bison, and turkey throughout the week. Shifting your focus to getting the right amounts of protein and fiber is also a sustainable way to protect your body from high LDL cholesterol and heart disease. It can also help with weight loss and maintaining a healthy weight. This combination's beautiful synergy contributes to fullness, energy balance, and satiation throughout the day.

Fat: The Misunderstood Macronutrient

After decades of fearing it, we're beginning to accept that eating some fat is essential for our health. Fat makes a difference by promoting more beneficial gut bacteria, lowering inflammation, and improving our hunger and fullness cues. Although necessary, not all fats are safe and healthy for cooking and eating. While there are fats that provide your body with anti-inflammatory properties, there are some that increase your disease risk and should be drastically reduced or avoided altogether.

Omega-3 Fatty Acids

Omega-3 fatty acids are a form of fat our body must get from food because it cannot make it on its own. They assist with many functions in the body, from brain health to maintaining healthy cholesterol levels. Omega-3 fatty acids help improve diversity among the microbes in our gut, particularly bifidobacterium, *Akkermansia muciniphila*, and lactobacillus.[17] Each of these microbes is known to improve digestion and the quality of mucus coating the gut lining. The downstream effect of having rich diversity in these bacteria is a better defense system starting in the gut, better nutrient absorption, and energy balance. Omega-3 fatty acids also prevent E. coli from overpopulating, and helps neutralize LPS which is a toxin found inside the bacterial film.

Omega-3s are primarily found in microalgae but are passed into fish when consumed. However, even if you don't eat meat or fish, you can still find foods to eat that are rich in omega-3 fatty acids. Including omega-3 fatty acids in your diet or supplementation is a helpful strategy to manage inflammation and support your gut health. There are eleven forms that omega-3 fatty acids come in, but eicosatetraenoic acid (EPA), docosahexaenoic acid (DHA), and docosapentaenoic acid (DPA) are the most potent for supporting a healthy gut. EPA decreases damage from toxins that interfere with the intestinal mucosa, acting as a defense mechanism. DHA plays a unique role in protecting the neurons in the gut and the brain, which communicate back and forth. DPA plays a firefighter role by using cytokine activity to lower inflammatory signaling between tissues and cells. A fantastic thing our bodies can do is convert EPA and DPA back and forth to each other, as long as we have enough of the original form. The human body can do the exact conversion between DPA and DHA to meet daily requirements. When looking for an omega-3 supplement, choose one that contains all three, EPA, DHA, and DPA, instead of just two forms. In one study, people who took an omega-3 supplement with all three included had a 63 percent increase in tissue levels as opposed to 41 percent taking a supplement with only DHA and EPA.[18]

Alpha-lipoic acid (ALA) is another form of omega-3 fatty acid that has a role in reducing inflammation, supporting glutathione activity, and mounting a more robust immune response.[19] Only 5 percent of ALA consumed can be converted into EPA and DHA, so ensure you eat foods rich in these fatty acids or take a quality fish oil supplement. The recommended guidelines for daily EPA and DHA omega-3 consumption is 250-3000 mg daily,[20] with a maximum safe dose of 5000 mg. While most people have the problem of not consuming enough omega-3 fatty acids, it is possible to get too many. Excess omega-3s have been linked with thinner blood, diabetes, and weight gain. Be especially mindful of chia seeds, as a two-table-spoon serving helps you reach that ceiling quickly. As with any supplement, check with your doctor before starting it to ensure it doesn't negatively interact with any medications you're taking. To help you in choosing foods to support your omega-3 needs, check the tables below and rotate these items into your diet throughout the month.

EPA-Rich Foods	DHA-Rich Foods
• Atlantic herring (3 oz = 770 mg) • Atlantic salmon (3 oz = 350 - 590 mg) • Sardines, canned (3 oz = 450 mg) • Atlantic mackerel (3 oz = 430 mg) • Oysters, wild (3 oz = 300 mg) • Salmon, canned (3 oz = 280 mg) • Sea bass (3 oz = 180 mg) • Shrimp, cooked (3 oz = 120 mg)	• Atlantic salmon, wild (3 oz = 1220 mg) • Atlantic herring (3 oz = 940 mg) • Sardines, canned (3 oz = 740 mg) • Salmon, canned (3 oz = 630 mg) • Atlantic mackerel (3 oz = 590 mg) • Sea bass (3 oz = 470 mg) • Oysters, wild (3 oz = 230 mg) • Shrimp, cooked (3 oz = 120 mg)

Table 3

DPA-Rich Foods	ALA-Rich Foods
• Atlantic salmon (3 oz = 340 mg) • Salmon, canned (3 oz = 170 mg) • Lamb (3 oz = 83 mg) • Mackerel (3 oz = 180 mg) • Grass-fed ground beef (3 oz = 65 mg)	• Chia seeds (1 oz = 5,000 mg) • Walnuts (1 oz = 2570 mg) • Whole flaxseeds (1 tbsp = 2350 mg) • Kidney beans, canned (½ cup = 100 mg)

Table 4

Omega-6 Fatty Acids – Polyunsaturated Fatty-Acids (PUFAS)

What is the scoop on omega-6s? Omega-6 fatty acids are a polyunsaturated fat (PUFA) source. These are considered healthy in the right amount and in whole-food form. They help supply energy to the body and produce and maintain healthy skin, hair, and bones. Omega-6 fatty acids are found in vegetable oils, salad dressings, and packaged foods. Walnuts, grapeseed oil, sunflower oil, pine nuts, soybean oil, almonds, tofu, and vegetable shortening are foods that are high in omega-6 fatty acids. Eating too many omega-6s (PUFAS) has been associated with obesity and increased inflammation. A possible reason for this is that they have longer fatty acid chains and are more likely to be stored as fat in the body rather than burned off for energy.[21] Monounsaturated fats (MUFAS) have shorter chains in their fatty acid structure and are easily consumed for energy, which you'll read about in a moment. One way to think of your omega-6 consumption is to eat them in ratio to omega-3 fatty acids. Unfortunately, the typical Western diet includes high levels of omega-6 fatty acids compared to omega-3s, at a ratio of 20:1.[22] Instead, consume foods with omega-3s and omega-6 fatty acids in a 2:1 ratio[23] to balance their helpful and anti-inflammatory properties.

The bottom line is that while omega-6 fatty acids are necessary for our health and longevity, most people eat too many. Eating more omega-6 fatty acids than needed can prevent the body from using the available omega-3s, which reduces or negates their anti-inflammatory nature.

INTEGRAL TIP: Rather than focusing primarily on the nutrition facts section or calories of each packaged food label, pay special attention to the ingredients list of each food. Most salad dressings, mayonnaise, and marinades are crafted with PUFAS as their base. The most common PUFAS you'll see are hydrogenated vegetable oil, sunflower oil, safflower oil, peanut oil, canola oil, corn oil, grapeseed oil, palm oil, and soybean oil. Some food brands have less inflammatory oils as their base. These are avocado, olive, coconut, and unrefined red palm oil.

Cod liver oil and flaxseed oil are also helpful, as they're rich in omega-3s.

Helpful Fat – Monounsaturated Fat (MUFAS)

Monounsaturated fats (MUFAS) are healthy fats that help protect your heart from disease by keeping low-density lipoprotein in a healthy range. To reap the benefits of monounsaturated fats in relation heart health, you should also lower your intake of inflammatory hydrogenated oils and trans-saturated fats in fast food, frozen food, and packaged food so the benefit is not canceled out. Monounsaturated fats come from avocados, nuts, flaxseed, pumpkin seeds, sesame seeds, olives, and olive oil.

Harmful Fats – Trans Fats

At first glance, a standard granola bar seems like an innocent and healthy choice, but when you read the ingredients label you'll notice that many are manufactured with trans-saturated fats. Trans-fats help increase the shelf life of products so they don't expire quickly. Unfortunately, the shelf life benefit of trans-fats has the opposite effect once inside the body. Trans-saturated fats, often seen as "partially hydrogenated" on ingredients lists, cause LDL to increase and simultaneously decrease HDL, the heart-protective fat. We need HDL to help clean our blood vessels and regulate our cholesterol. Lowering HDL lowers cholesterol in an unhelpful way, which increases the risk for heart attacks and plaque formation.

<u>Harmful or Helpful Fat – Saturated Fats</u>

Saturated fats are hugely debated in the medical, nutrition, and health sciences. For the longest time, many believed that all saturated fats increase LDL, harming your heart and increasing your risk for heart disease. Then, new studies began to emerge that suggested controversial evidence. One of the richest sources of saturated fat from meat is beef. Meat from grass-fed cows contains fatty acids with a higher antioxidant profile and more precursors to vitamins A and E[24] and glutathione, a potent antioxidant known to fight cancer cells and support the immune system. Additionally, grass-fed beef is a source of omega-3 fatty acids, which we know reduce inflammation and must be a part of our diet if we want to protect our bodies from chronic diseases.

In 2021, a study unveiled that the U.S. Dietary Guidelines for reducing saturated fat as a strategy for reducing heart disease and heart attacks don't actually follow evidence.[25] Reducing saturated fat intake does not consistently translate to the reduction of heart disease in the studies. We need to debunk the belief that eating saturated fat always contributes to an increased risk of heart disease and see that we don't need to eliminate these fat sources from our lives to be well. Saturated fat can be part of a healthy diet if it comes from a suitable source. Organic coconuts, dairy products, and pasture-raised, 100-percent grass-fed, grass-finished meats are the purest and highest quality saturated fat sources.

How Certain Foods Affect Gut Health

What's clear among all the dietary theories is one common denominator: whole, unrefined foods have a powerful effect on healing the body. If you can increase the amount of whole, nutrient-dense foods in your diet, you are on the right path to healing and reaching any sustainable weight loss goals. Should we eat processed, packaged foods, including refined carbs? Processed carbohydrates don't offer a rich nutrient profile and are often unfilling and leave us wanting more. Refined carbs should not be labeled as "bad," but I encourage you to look at these foods with curiosity and ask what amount of them is honoring to your body and the unique healing journey you are on.

Take this a step further by discovering any food sensitivities and eliminating them. This will help you have even better results with skin, digestion, and weight balance. It is possible to improve your body's response to foods by going through a healing process, which you will find outlined in chapter 8.

GRAINS

The controversy over grains has been hard to keep up with. While some sources claim they are inflammatory and should have no place in our diets, others state that the fiber and carbohydrate content inside grains is necessary for a healthy diet and digestion. Remember that no body is created equal, and grains affect each person differently. Whole versus refined grains also digest differently, making us feel energetic or sluggish.

Refined grains, like wheat flour, are milled down to small particles for the purpose of baking. A whole grain is less processed, and grains like quinoa, brown rice, and barley are in their whole-food form. When the body begins digesting a meal containing whole grains, it's a long process. The stomach acid takes longer to break down each grain, and the carbohydrates are converted to glucose slowly compared to refined carbohydrates.

For refined carbohydrates, most commonly found in processed and packaged foods, the macronutrient profile might look the same on the packaging, but something different is happening on the inside of the body during digestion. The carbohydrates are already broken down into a minimal, refined form, and the blood glucose rises very quickly as the food is digested. Looking at an Oreo cookie, for example, three cookies contain twenty-five grams of carbohydrates, fourteen grams coming from sugar and high fructose corn syrup, and no fiber. The rest of the carbohydrates come from unbleached, enriched wheat flour modified to reduce iron and increase B vitamins. Compare this with a serving of old-fashioned oats. A half-cup serving of old-fashioned oats contains twenty-seven grams of carbohydrates, four grams of fiber, and one gram of sugar. Though providing similar energy numbers from carbohydrates, the difference between oats and the Oreo cookie is that once the oats are digesting, it brings a sense of fullness from the fibers in the whole grains and the bulk of the food. Oats will provide stable, slow-release energy, while Oreos will instantly release their carbohydrate load. Knowing this helps you understand which carbohydrates are best for you and your goals. Suppose your goal is to heal your gut and lose weight. In this case, the old-fashioned oats are a better choice overall. The fiber content provides food to gut microbes, helps digestion, helps you feel full, keeps energy levels stable, and makes you feel satisfied for a longer period of time. Additionally, the original B vitamins are left intact and haven't been re-added to make up for what is lost in food processing. The low sugar content can contribute to a healthy balance of candida, as some gut imbalances include candida overgrowth.

GLUTEN: Should You Eat It?

Gluten is another element of food that has become controversial, and you may be wondering whether you should eliminate it from your diet. The correct answer is that it's up to you and your body's unique needs. While it affects some people severely, gluten causes small levels of damage to the intestinal tract when it's digested.[26] The best strategy regarding gut health and gluten is to drastically reduce the amount you eat or eliminate it from your diet. In my case, gluten makes me bloat slightly. However, I didn't realize this until after I did an elimination protocol removing gluten and reintroducing it later. Eliminating gluten for six months gave me valuable information about how my body reacts to it, which I never would have had if I had not tried removing it.

VEGETABLES

Vegetables seem to be tolerated differently by each person. For one person, eating more vegetables will help support the liver's natural detoxification, weight loss, and improvement in diseases like diabetes. However, another person might experience the worst abdominal pain and bloating of their life when eating vegetables such as broccoli or onion due to their specific fibers. This is where it's important to highlight how an elimination diet and food sensitivity testing can fill in the gray areas where you're feeling mystified. While it's true that vegetables are a healthy source of fiber and nutrients, there are unique individuals who should be avoiding many, if not all, vegetables due to the situation in their gut. It's possible the gut tissue can be too damaged from inflammatory bowel disease to comfortably and properly digest vegetables. Thankfully, with intentional healing and working closely with a provider who understands the gut, you can regain your ability to digest veggies.

Legumes

Are they great for gut health, or are they garbage? Generally, this comes down to a person's ability to digest them. However, many people report improved digestion from eating beans as part of their daily diet. If you choose to do an elimination diet to see how beans affect you, remember that the body has to get used to digesting them again, so slowly introducing them back in once you've taken them out for a time is an intelligent strategy. Start with a few bites and gradually increase the amount to a regular serving size of 1/2 cup.

Is it a coincidence that many cultures experiencing longevity include beans as a staple in their diets? Lets zoom in for a closer look. Eating beans can protect your heart, help improve insulin resistance, and support the liver's detox process.[27] Eating beans daily helps with hormone balance and reducing triglycerides. The soluble fiber in beans binds to excess hormone components and triglycerides, helping them exit through stool. Otherwise, they would be recycled and reabsorbed into the body. Additionally, because of the fiber content and ability to support our blood sugar and insulin response, many people find beans to be a helpful food for maintaining a healthy weight.

Also, beans become more easily digestible when pressure cooked and the lectins are removed. Lectins have a resilient structure and will not break down unless cooked at temperatures higher than one hundred degrees Celsius for longer than thirty minutes.[28] Lectins are a carbohydrate-binding protein found in some foods and have been known to cause digestive issues such as bloating and pain. Someone lectin-sensitive might experience bloating or digestive pain, but the issue goes deeper. Brain fog, fatigue, and a general not-well feeling can result from the lectins' systemic effect that can adversely influence inflammation and the immune system. When studied in animals, lectins were found to be attracted to the gut lining, or epithelium, and can sometimes prevent the absorption of nutrients. Research suggests that kidney beans have a more bothersome type of lectin that some suspect is the reason for many reported cases of food poisoning after eating them. Foods that are highest in lectins are legumes (beans, lentils, peas, soybeans, peanuts), nightshade vegetables (eggplant, tomato, potato, bell pepper), and grains.

This doesn't mean we need to eliminate these foods forever, but it helps us to be aware when we eat foods with high lectin content. As you consume them, notice how you feel and if you're having any symptoms, digestive or other.

Fruits

Fruit is rich in minerals, vitamins, antioxidants, and prebiotic fibers. Prebiotic fibers help feed the good microbes in our gut, therefore allowing the gut to heal and the microbiome to flourish. Fruit was discovered to lower the risk for type 2 diabetes, possibly due to the fiber and nutrient content in addition to the carbohydrates and sugar. Fruit is generally considered nourishing to the gut and to be part of a balanced diet. Some of the best fruits for gut health include berries, bananas, grapefruit, watermelon, and apples.

Dairy

Milk, cheese, and other dairy products are rich in protein, calcium, magnesium, potassium, phosphorus, zinc, and B vitamins.[29] Although nutritious and with the ability to genuinely contribute to better health in many individuals, there are a few things to know about milk-based foods that may influence your decision to include them in your diet.

The original purpose of milk is for baby mammals to have a source of nutrients to grow and become strong and healthy. In cow's milk—the variety most people consume in the United States—there's a protein called casein, which breaks down into a compound called casomorphin. This substance behaves similarly to morphine in the brain, causing addictive feelings in a person. In a baby calf, casomorphin is critical in helping the baby mammal remain "hooked" on the mother's milk for as long as it needs to grow and thrive. But for human adults, we don't benefit from casomorphin in the same way, and it may have an adverse effect that challenges our ability to eat dairy in moderation.

Additionally, many people find that they are sensitive to the components in dairy. Lactose, the sugar in milk and dairy products, can cause bloating and digestive discomfort if you're sensitive to it. Whey and casein, the proteins in milk, are common culprits for bloating and intolerance. If you suspect you have a sensitivity to dairy, you can get your blood tested or have muscle testing done to uncover which components of dairy are most bothersome. In addition to testing, you can dial into your individual needs even further by going through an elimination protocol for three to six months. Remove the foods you are sensitive to and systematically add particular versions of that food back in. For instance, if you were tested for intolerances to dairy and your test showed that you were sensitive to whey, you could take all dairy products out of your diet for at least six weeks and reintroduce ghee first and sheep's milk cheese second. (You can find more resources on effectively going through an elimination protocol in chapter 8.) While an elimination diet may sound like the last thing you're interested in doing and perhaps even unrealistic, I share from personal experience that it is 100 percent worth your time, discipline, and effort. Imagine doing the difficult thing for three to six months and allowing your gut to heal. Then, following the elimination phase, your reward is a lifetime of understanding what your body thrives on and also what it doesn't tolerate very well. This respite from foods that are inflaming you allows your body to heal and become more acute in noticing what makes you feel "off." You'll have a super-sense about the provoking food culprits you've had in your diet for years. This is nearly impossible to achieve without going through an elimination diet.

Sugars

Earlier in this chapter, we discussed how refined sugar might encourage dysbiosis and an overgrowth of candida.[30] Sugar is a demonized subject in our diets. Accused of being addictive like cocaine and a leading culprit for obesity, it's no wonder many people say things like "I'm being bad right now" after eating a couple Girl Scout cookies. Sugar has gotten enough attention to deserve its own chapter, perhaps even its own book. It's not that sugar itself is inherently bad, it's the way that we're consuming it. For instance, the sugar content in a banana or an apple is accompanied by fibers, vitamins, and minerals to support many functions and needs of our body. When you juice the fruit and remove the fibers, you're also removing an important component that helps regulate blood sugar (fiber), and it results in blood sugar spikes. Soda, bottled juices, and coffee are drinks that many people have multiple times per day. It might not seem significant because it's just a drink, but this is a big issue. The daily recommendation of maximum sugar intake from the American Heart Association is twenty-four grams for women and thirty-six grams for men. This is about nine to ten teaspoons. Looking at the table below, you can see how drinking just one bottle of Gatorade brings you up to that maximum.

Drink	Grams of Sugar	Teaspoons of Sugar
Gatorade (Grape flavor) 600 ml	36	9
Starbucks Frappuccino (Grande – 16 oz)	59	15
Coca-Cola (375 ml – 1 can)	40	9.5

Table 5

Across the globe, we've been eating and drinking way more added sugar than is healthy for us. The irony is that many sugar-laden foods and drinks have an attractively low price, but the cost is poor health, which becomes expensive and time-consuming as you visit doctor after doctor, pay for your insurance, medications, and trips to the hospital for medical issues. The most often heard argument is that eating better food is just too expensive. Unfortunately, the price that many people pay in the long run for regular and high consumption of refined, high-sugar foods ends up being more expensive due to the cost of having medical issues. Sugar consumption hasn't only increased in high-income countries in the past ten to twenty years; medium and low-income countries are now consuming much more sugar than before,[31] which is a considerable issue because it causes such a burden on the health of individuals. Obesity, diabetes, and tooth decay might be the first things that come to mind, but sugar plays a dominating role in digestive, metabolic, and heart diseases as well. Our brain, digestive, and heart health depend on us developing a balanced relationship with sugar intake.

How do you go about reducing your sugar intake when sugar is tucked away in more foods than you could have ever guessed? Read articles and books like this and begin intentionally scanning labels to educate yourself on what products you're purchasing that have unexpected added sugar. Low-fat yogurt, dressings, barbecue sauce, ketchup, sports drinks, juices, spaghetti sauce, soups, granola, and chocolate milk are several foods that have a sneaky and surprising amount of added sugars in them. Looking at figure 21, you can see how many grams of added sugar are inside a well-known brands of nonfat yogurt.

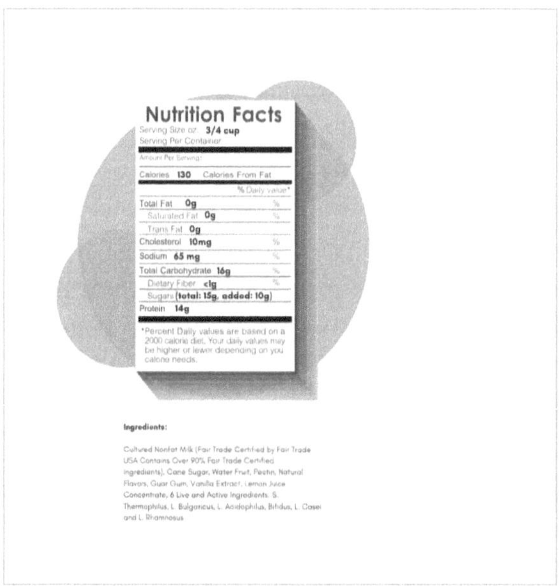

Figure 21

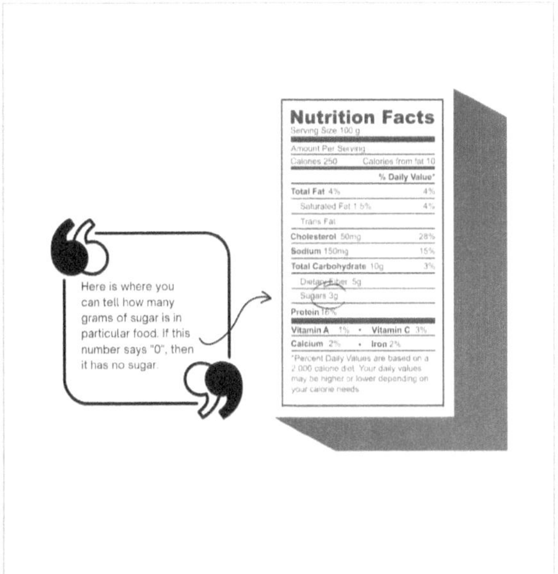

Figure 22

LOOKING at the first figure and reading the label (the nutrition facts and the ingredients section), you can see that the total amount of sugar in ¾ cup of yogurt is fifteen grams, and the added sugar brings in ten grams. That means five grams come from naturally occurring sugar before cane sugar was added, and the other ten grams of added sugar mostly come from the cane sugar, then pectin. Some labels will have it listed as "added sugar" outright, while other labels are harder to read. If you're unsure if something has added sugar, another way to check is to read the ingredients list section underneath the label. The most commonly seen added sugars are listed in bold lettering below.

Common Forms of Added Sugar on Ingredients Labels:

• **Dextrose**	• Crystalline fructose	• Treacle
• **Fructose**	• **Date sugar**	• Beet sugar
• **Galactose**	• Demerara sugar	• **Brown sugar**
• **Glucose**	• Dextrin	• Cane juice crystals
• **Lactose**	• Golden sugar	• **Cane sugar**
• **Maltose**	• Confectioners' sugar	• Castor sugar
• **Sucrose**	• **Corn syrup solids**	• **Coconut sugar**
• **Maltodextrin**	• **Agave nectar/syrup**	• Carob syrup
• Glucose syrup solids	• Barley malt	• **Corn syrup**
• Icing sugar	• Blackstrap molasses	• **Evaporated cane juice**
• Grape sugar	• **Brown rice syrup**	• **Fruit juice**
• Panela sugar	• Buttered sugar	• Golden syrup
• **Raw sugar**	• Buttercream	• Invert sugar
• Muscovado sugar	• **Granulated sugar**	• **Maple syrup**
• Sorghum syrup	• **Turbinado sugar**	• **Rice syrup**
	• Yellow sugar	• Refiner's syrup

Table 6

Some of the listed items don't **seem** to have a name indicating added sugar. Sorghum syrup, **dextrin**, and barley malt don't exactly trigger a realization of "hey, that's sugar," but they're in a lot of our food. This is why I **suspect** so many people take in added sugars without even **questioning** it. How to decipher ingredients labels and nutrition facts will be one of the most helpful tools for you when you're learning how to reduce added sugars in your daily lifestyle. Applying what you discover will save your brain, heart, and gut.

Probiotic Foods

There are a variety of plant-based and animal-based probiotic foods. Probiotic foods contain live cultures of bacteria that help support gut health and digestion. They are rich in many vitamins and minerals, which adds to their value. Whether or not you are taking a probiotic supplement, there will always be a benefit to including probiotic foods as well. When yogurt, sauerkraut, and kombucha are made, they can have a wide variety of probiotic strains that support various areas of the body. Interestingly, the probiotic quality of yogurt makes it easier to digest for some who are normally sensitive to dairy. Raw probiotic foods have the most nutrient-dense profile because they have not been heated through pasteurization.

PROBIOTIC FOODS LIST

- Kimchi (fermented cabbage with spices originating from Korea)
- Sauerkraut
- Lassi (a probiotic yogurt drink originating from India)
- Kefir
- Refrigerator pickles
- Natto (fermented soybeans dish originating from Japan)
- Yogurt
- Tempeh
- Miso
- Tofu
- Kombucha
- Gouda, mozzarella, and cheddar cheese
- Feta cheese
- Fermented vegetables

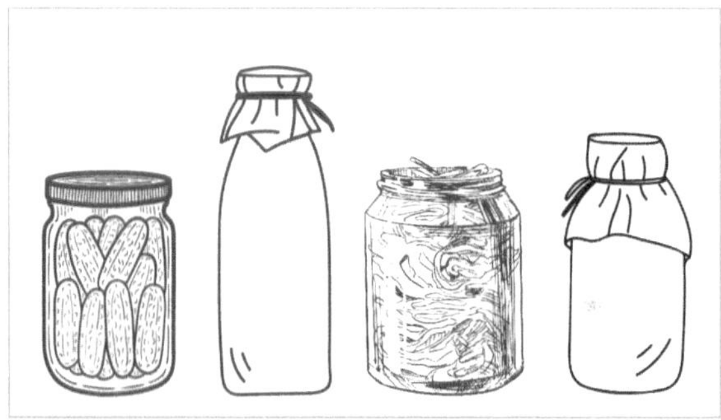

Figure 23

FODMAP

What is FODMAP? FODMAP stands for fermentable oligosaccharides, disaccharides, monosaccharides, and polyols. Polyol refers to sugar alcohols. Common sugar alcohols are sorbitol, mannitol, and xylitol. In the simplest terms, FODMAP foods are those that are made up of sugars that the intestines do not absorb very well. Not everyone will react to these sugars, but in some people, FODMAP-rich foods cause symptoms of painful gas, bloating, constipation, and diarrhea. Reducing or eliminating them for a time has helped many understand their body's intolerances. Foods that fall under the FODMAP category are dairy products, products containing gluten (bread, crackers, cereals), beans and other legumes, artichokes, asparagus, onions, garlic, and some fruits, such as apples, pears, cherries, and peaches.

Usually, digestive enzymes break food components down to be readily absorbed by the small intestine. The pancreas and other digestive organs release digestive enzymes after eating. Still, amylase can't break down the sugar chains in high FODMAP foods, resulting in these compounds making their way through the small intestine undigested. When undigested food particles make it to the colon, it causes gastrointestinal distress. Not all FODMAPs trigger the same digestive symptoms in people with IBS, and these foods may cause pain for those without IBS as well. Eating a slice of bread itself may not trigger an IBS flare-up, but consuming a slice bread with cheese, a glass of milk, and an apple could cause a combination of painful symptoms for someone who struggles with FODMAP intolerance.[32] These foods also feed bacteria, which may work against you if you're trying to heal SIBO.

A low-FODMAP diet means that you reduce or eliminate the foods that are high in FODMAPs and focus on eating foods that have the least number of bothersome components. Foods lower in FODMAPs are eggs, meat, feta cheese, rice, quinoa, oats, potato, tomato, cucumber, zucchini, grapes, oranges, berries, pineapple, and almonds. While engaging in a low-FODMAP protocol can be helpful for many struggling with IBS, the downfalls can be difficulty sticking with it long-term, nutritional deficiencies, and cost. Since a low-FODMAP diet is restrictive and requires a lot of food elimination, the best thing you can do is work closely with a health expert like a nutritionist to ensure you're meeting your nutrient requirements while following the protocol. You can learn more about nutritionists who are qualified in this area in the resources section in the back of this book.

KEY TAKEAWAYS

Dialing in your nutrition is necessary to your success in having a healthy gut and healing your body. As we wrap up the longest chapter in this book, here are the key takeaways from this chapter to help hone your focus.

- **Eat fibrous, whole-food carbohydrates.** Pair them with protein and fat for higher satiation value, the sensation of fullness, and sustainable energy.

- **Get prebiotic and probiotic foods in your daily** to support healthy gut bacteria.
- **Eat a moderate protein diet balanced with fiber.** Aim to get twenty to thirty grams of protein and seven to twelve grams of fiber per meal. If you struggle with bloating after eating fibrous foods, work to slowly increase these foods to allow your gut microbes and gut to adjust to them.
- **Don't aim to cut out a food group permanently.** Removing fats, dairy, sugar, carbs, and FODMAPs permanently or even for extended periods will impact your body's hormone and homeostatic functions. Additionally, this can place stress on the body and play a role in nutritional requirements not being met. This can manifest as irregular or lost menstrual cycles in women, weight loss resistance, low energy, hormone imbalances, and depression. Eating disorders may develop as well.
- **Approach food with a dual focus.** Balance your future goals with your current gut and metabolic health. Challenge what you've accepted for "truth" in knowledge about health and taking care of your body. This especially applies to weight loss and dieting.
- **It's not just sugar or hydrogenated oils that cause poor health.** It's an amalgamation of eating multiple foods containing these ingredients—such as sugary cereals, sodas, fast food, and packaged food—that are causing it. In addition, stress, lack of sleep, dehydration, and consumption of alcohol, drugs, and caffeine will increase poor health outcomes.
- **Avoid extreme diets or programs offering fast solutions.**
- **Replace sugars with nonglycemic sweeteners such as allulose, monk fruit extract, and stevia.** Sugar from

fruit, honey, coconut, and dates will still raise the blood sugar but will also offer support to the liver and adrenal glands in small amounts and are the healthiest choices regarding added sugars.

- **Spend time reading and learning how to decipher nutrition labels and ingredient lists.** This is a critical piece in your ability to recognize where inflammatory fats and added sugars in your food choices are coming from.
- **Choose beneficial fats that decrease inflammation, protect your heart, and heal your gut.** Drastically reduce or eliminate inflammatory, harmful fats:
- Trans-Saturated Fats – Hydrogenated oils and margarine, most often found in fast food, frozen meals, and shelf-stable packaged foods. These are the most toxic and harmful to our heart health.
- PUFAS (Polyunsaturated Fats) – Canola, soybean, and other seed oils that are typically found in dressings, marinades, packaged foods, and other condiments.
- Commercially-Raised and Processed Saturated Fats – From nonorganic, commercially-raised cows and farmed sources. Consume a moderate amount of saturated fats from grass-fed animal products (beef, butter, ghee, tallow, lard, coconut) for the best health outcomes.

8

FOOD ALLERGIES, INTOLERANCES, AND SENSITIVITIES

Twenty percent of the world's population struggles with reactions to food. While bringing food's influence on the microbiome into the light, it's essential to note the differences between food allergies, intolerances, and sensitivities.

Food allergies involve a severe immune response that happens when you ingest or come into contact with a particular food. The immune system releases an antibody called immunoglobulin E (IgE). In some cases, an allergy is so severe that being close to the food can cause anaphylactic shock. This allergic reaction is life-threatening because tissues in the trachea can swell and block off oxygen to the lungs and the rest of the body.

Food intolerances do not involve the immune system but manifest as difficulty digesting certain foods due to not being able to break down the components. Lactose intolerance is a common example of a food sensitivity. Lactose is a sugar found in milk and dairy products. If someone is lactose intolerant, they have a deficiency of the digestive enzyme lactase, which is produced in our small intestine.[1] Dairy cannot be adequately broken down when eaten due to lactase enzyme deficiency. This results in abdominal pain, bloating, and gas. The undigested food particles get pushed along to the colon, where the gut bacteria attempt to break the particles down by fermentation, which causes more gas. The colon can sometimes flood to dilute the undigested food, resulting in diarrhea. Usually, lactic acid bacteria, such as lactobacillus and bifidobacterium, help with the breakdown of lactose and create the byproduct lactic acid. Lactic acid does not give us any nutritional benefit, nor does it cause bloating or abdominal pain. This quick look at how lactic acid bacteria help digestion shows how adding fermented foods to your diet or taking a probiotic with lactic acid bacteria could improve your digestion.

Food sensitivities are different from food allergies because they are not life-threatening and don't involve a severe response from the immune system. Even though discovering your food sensitivities is one of the best ways to decrease chronic, low-grade inflammation and feel your absolute best, some people can go through their entire lives without knowing they have a food sensitivity. The immune system releases immunoglobulin G (IgG) or immunoglobulin A (IgA) antibodies when a food you're sensitive to enters your digestive tract. What most people are unaware of is that consuming foods you're sensitive to can also spike your blood sugar levels, even if the food is low-glycemic, which is a "survival response" the body goes through in the inflammatory process.[2] This is where continuous glucose monitors can be helpful, as they give you real-time data about your blood sugar after you consume certain foods. Elevated blood sugar levels from consuming your food sensitivities can contribute to chronic, low-grade inflammation and stress over time.

Histamine and gluten sensitivities are also quite common. Foods that are high in histamine or histamine-releasers are:

- Alcohol
- Canned foods
- Some matured cheeses
- Some meats (i.e., shellfish, salami, ham, meat with nitrates)
- Chickpeas
- Soy
- Nuts (i.e., peanuts, cashews)
- Chocolate
- Ready-made meals (i.e., frozen meals)
- Artificial preservatives and food dyes
- Citrus fruits
- Tomatoes
- Wheat germ
- Benzoate (a preservative found in packaged food and cosmetics)
- Sulfites (found in packaged meats and some wine)
- Glutamate (commonly found in monosodium glutamate, or MSG).[3]

HAVING a gluten sensitivity makes it harder to digest gluten, a protein found in wheat, barley, and rye. Being sensitive to histamine foods means you are deficient in diamine oxidase, the enzyme that helps break it down. Protease and amylase are enzymes responsible for digesting gluten, and they are produced in the stomach, pancreas, and small intestine. Celiac disease is different from gluten sensitivity because it is an autoimmune disease that triggers an immune response, damaging the small intestine. Without diagnosis and treatment of celiac disease, the small intestine can become permanently damaged, and the body will not be able to absorb nutrients properly.[4] Common symptoms of celiac disease are vomiting, mouth ulcers, seizures, diarrhea, itchy skin, headaches, fatigue, bone and joint pain, acid reflux, confusion, and weight loss. If you're experiencing any of these symptoms and the reason is so far unexplained, visit a doctor and specialist soon.

It's important to address any food sensitivities you may have because if you continue to eat food your body is sensitive to, it will cause chronic, low-grade inflammation in your body and the gut. Persistent inflammation prevents your gut from healing and regenerating healthy cells, and will cause an increase in leaky gut. Keep a food diary when you suspect you might be sensitive to certain foods. Writing down what you're eating and any symptoms that pop up becomes critical in exposing foods that cause a disruption in your body. The following actions can also help reveal food sensitivities.

VISIT a Holistic or Functional Practitioner in Your Area

A holistic or functional practitioner can usually order a comprehensive blood panel that will give you a list of your food sensitivities, graded between nonexistent, mild, moderate, and severe. These tests give the most information on food sensitivities and allergies, but they also tend to be the most expensive. Expect to pay anywhere from $300 to $1000 for a comprehensive blood allergy panel.

Additionally, some providers are trained in applied kinesiology (muscle testing) for detecting food sensitivities. Muscle testing is not scientifically proven for diagnostic purposes for allergies, and it's important to notice that food allergies require more caution than a suspected sensitivity.[5] If you suspect you have a food allergy, visit your primary doctor. Proven tests for diagnosing food allergies are oral food challenges, skin prick tests, IgE blood testing, and food elimination diets.[6] However, muscle testing can certainly be helpful when navigating sensitivities. In a review of twelve muscle-testing randomized control trials (RCTs), this testing was found to be useful for clinical practice.[7] However, it does seem that to be scientifically proven, muscle-testing for the diagnosis of food allergies would need to go through more technical testing methods. The recommendations and plans based on muscle testing and follow-up reassessment results have been effective for me, my friends, my family, and my clientele.

Do a Food Elimination Diet

A food elimination diet is one of the best methods for understanding your food sensitivities. You can also remove them from your diet for ninety days at a minimum and reintroduce them one by one.[8] I once did an elimination diet after spending a little over three years recovering from my eating disorder, which helped me heal my digestive system and metabolism even more. While it's not easy or fun because of the level of discipline it takes to stick with it, the results of a successfully done elimination protocol can give you the best, most specific answers about your food sensitivities. Discovering my food sensitivities and taking them out resulted in better energy, better gut and digestive health, weight balance, and a happier relationship with food.

If you're recovering from disordered eating patterns, it's essential to understand where you are in your relationship with food. Elimination diets are highly restrictive and can trigger intense cravings and binge-eating episodes if you aren't getting enough calories and nutrients from the foods on your protocol. If you have not spent enough time healing your mind and body after the disorder, you may not be ready for a food elimination diet, which can do more harm than good if you are still in the recovery process. Here are the steps to a successful food elimination diet:

- Completely eliminate trigger foods for three weeks. If you're not sure what your trigger foods are, you can follow the list in figure 23.
- At the end of three weeks, reintroduce one food at a time, eating one to three small portions of that food during the next three days. Take note of any symptoms you experience during each food reintroduction. The goal is to reintroduce a new food every four days.

- Repeat this until you've tried reintroducing all foods but leave out any foods that caused a trigger in symptoms. For example, during the reintroduction process, if you notice a rash appear and mouth itchiness when eating eggs, that is a sign you're sensitive to eggs and they should be removed as you continue to reintroduce foods.

You can find a helpful symptom-tracking resource in the bonus PDF.

Foods to Avoid on an Elimination Diet	Foods That You Can Eat on an Elimination Diet
• **Caffeine sources** (coffee, sodas, black tea, green tea)	• **Most fruits and vegetables,** except for citrus fruits and nightshade vegetables
• **Nightshade vegetables** (eggplant, bell peppers, white potato, many spices, tomato)	• **Grains:** White and brown rice, buckwheat
• **Nuts and seeds**	• **Meat:** turkey, game salmon and other cold-water fish (salmon)
• **Gluten, wheat, and starchy foods** such as rye, millet, and oats	• **Coconut products** (coconut milk, oil, and flour)
• **Some meat** (eggs, chicken, shellfish, beef, cold-cuts, salami)	• Olive oil and flaxseed oil
• **Dairy products** (cheese, milk, yogurt)	• Water and herbal tea
• **Legumes** (beans, lentils)	• **Fresh herbs,** spices (except for pepper and paprika), and apple cider vinegar
• **Butter,** margarine, hydrogenated oils, mayonnaise	
• **Sauces,** mustard, relish, and ketchup	
• **Sugar, honey, maple syrup** and all other sources of sugar (a complete list can be found in Chapter 7)	
• **Citrus fruits** such as lemons, oranges, and grapefruits	

Figure 23 - Reference: See Rakul, D. (2018) for more information on elimination diets.

It's never a bad idea to work with a professional when doing an elimination diet. Functional medicine, holistic and integrative medical doctors, nutritionists, and coaches are professionals who can help guide you through an elimination protocol while meeting your nutritional requirements. A list of nutrition and provider resources is in the back of this book, as well as a website you can use to locate a functional medicine provider near you.

· · ·

Key Takeaways:

- Food allergies involve a severe immune response that happens when you ingest or come into contact with a particular food.
- Food intolerances do not involve the immune system but manifest as difficulty digesting certain foods due to not being able to break down the components.
- Food sensitivities are not life-threatening and don't involve a severe response from the immune system.
- Uncovering your food sensitivities with an elimination diet or testing help you target additional sources of inflammation.

9

PROBIOTICS AND SUPPLEMENTS FOR GUT HEALTH

P robiotics are microorganisms that are cultured from a source (human, animal, dairy, or plant) and can be found in foods or manufactured into a capsule or pill form.

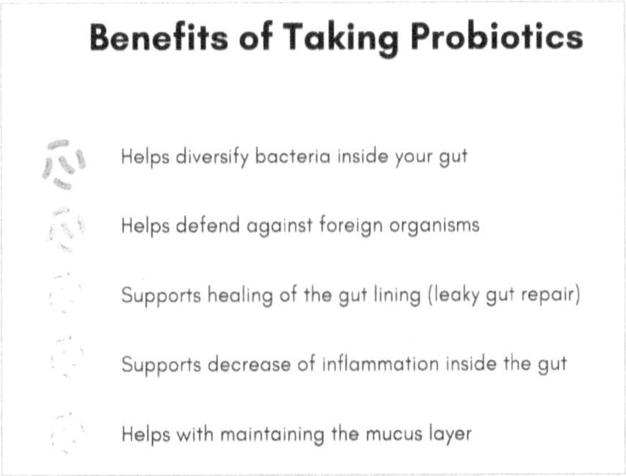

Benefits of Taking Probiotics

Helps diversify bacteria inside your gut

Helps defend against foreign organisms

Supports healing of the gut lining (leaky gut repair)

Supports decrease of inflammation inside the gut

Helps with maintaining the mucus layer

Figure 24 - Reference: See Sanders, M. E. (2011) for more information on the benefits of probiotics

PREBIOTICS ARE nutrients that supply probiotic bacteria with food and energy to create byproducts that provide benefits.[1] Synbiotics are a combination of both prebiotics and probiotics.[2]

On the back of a probiotic supplement's packaging, you'll notice that the names of the bacteria are broken up, designating the family, species, and strain. Each probiotic contains different strains and counts of bacteria and provides different benefits when ingested. When selecting the probiotic, choosing one with an enteric coating, which acts as a surrounding suit of armor that keeps the bacteria from being killed by stomach acid and will ensure that the maximum living dose arrives to your colon. Another kind of probiotic that has a protective coating ensuring lively probiotic delivery is known as "spore-based" probiotics. The colony forming-units (CFU) tell us how potent a probiotic is.

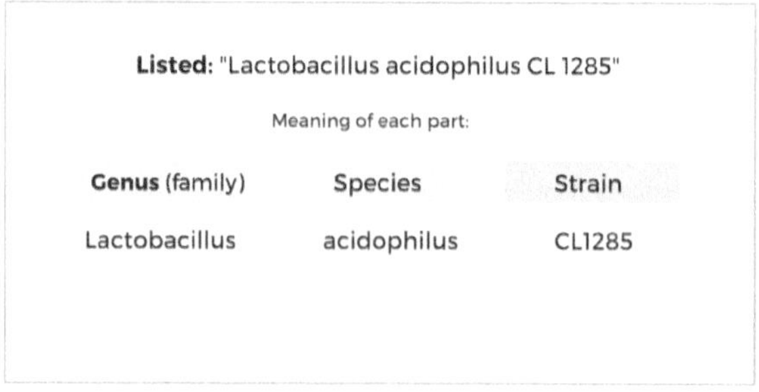

Figure 25

In order for probiotics to give health benefits, the bacteria need to be alive and taken in large enough doses to be effective.[3] It's important to do some research before taking a probiotic supplement to ensure that the strains inside have some research behind them regarding what you're trying to improve about your gut health. For example, *Lactobacillus casei* and *Lactobacillus acidophilus* species and strains were found to be effective in improving diarrhea as a symptom of SIBO.[4] Many lactobacillus species and strains have been found to be helpful in relieving clostridium difficile infections as well as the inflammatory bowel diseases ulcerative colitis and Crohn's disease.[5] In following a regimen of probiotics, including strains of *Bacillus clausii,* people had normal hydrogen breath tests, showing results that were just as effective as antibiotics. Industrialized countries are noticing that a bacteria called *Bifidobacterium longum infantis* (B. infantis), naturally occurring in babies, is decreasing due to antibiotic use and higher incidence of C-sections. This strain helps decrease intestinal inflammation in some babies by 55 percent.[6] *Saccharomyces boulardii,* a naturally occurring yeast and a common yeast strain in probiotic supplements, can support reduction of inflammation in the GI tract and overgrown candida fungi.[7]

Species and Strains of Probiotics That Support Specific Issues

IBS

- *Lactobacillus bulgaricus*
- *Lactobacillus lactis*
- *Streptococcus thermophilus*
- *Bifidobacterium infantis 35624*
- *Lactobacillus rhamnosus GG*
- *Lactobacillus plantarum*

Stress, Mood, Mental Functioning

- *Bifidobacterium Longum Rosell - 175 and B. Longum 1714*
- *Lactobacillus acidophilus Rosell-52*
- *Lactobacillus casei Shirota*

Diarrhea

- *Lactobacillus reuteri protectis SD2112*
- *Saccharomyces boulardii*

Figure 26 - Reference: See Ciorba M. A. (2012) for more Information on strains specific for IBS, Bercik, P. (2011) for more Information on Bifidobacterium longum and stress, and Wilkins (2018) for more Information on lactobacillus species.

SOMETHING that many people don't know about probiotics is that most of the bacteria inside don't actually seed into the GI tract and become permanent residents of your microbiome.[8] They help by supporting a need while they are there, similar to a traveling businessperson, but they exit in one to four weeks[9] and most don't colonize permanently. Some may actually become part of the microbial family; however, the most likely microorganism to colonize are those from the lactobacillus family. Lactobacillus were found to have a special protein that helps them adhere to our gastrointestinal layer.[10] [11]

You'll know a probiotic is working if you're experiencing regularity in digestion and bowel activity and reduction of symptoms you had before. Studies have show that people who supplemented with a probiotic noticed improvement in GERD, or acid reflux.[12] You can find a list of recommended probiotic brands in the Resources section in the back of this book.

Collagen

Collagen is a protein source that is sourced from the bones, ligament and cartilage of animals. It's helpful for gut health because it contains high levels of amino acids glycine, glutamine, and proline which support healthy connective tissue development for the gut and skin.[13] Supplementing with 20 grams of collagen daily was found to help reduce bloating in women.[14] The best ways to get collagen daily are by consuming bone broth, a supplement powder, or powdered gelatin.

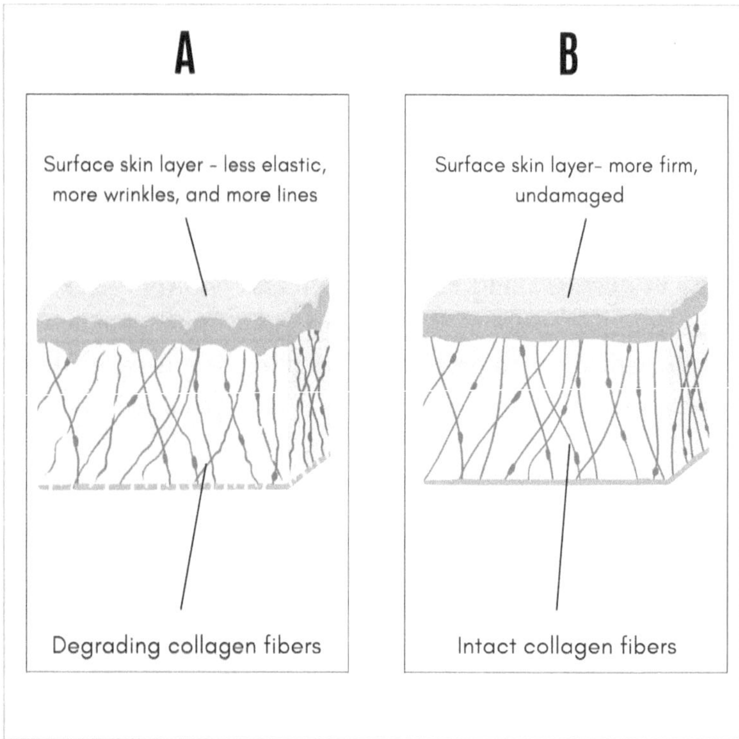

Figure 27

L-glutamine

Glutamine is an amino acid that plays a role in regulating the intestinal barrier and supporting the immune system.[15] Research for proving glutamine's usefulness in healing leaky gut is still in process, but many people report drastic improvement in gut-related symptoms after supplementing with this amino acid. You can purchase L-glutamine in a dissolvable powder. L-glutamine is tasteless, making it easy to add it to smoothies or mix it into a glass of water.

Aloe Vera

Aloe Vera leaf has a compound called aloin inside its gel and juice that acts as a natural antibacterial. [16] Aloe Vera helps keep gut bacteria in balance and supports digestion by regulating enzyme release. It's also been used as a remedy for constipation.

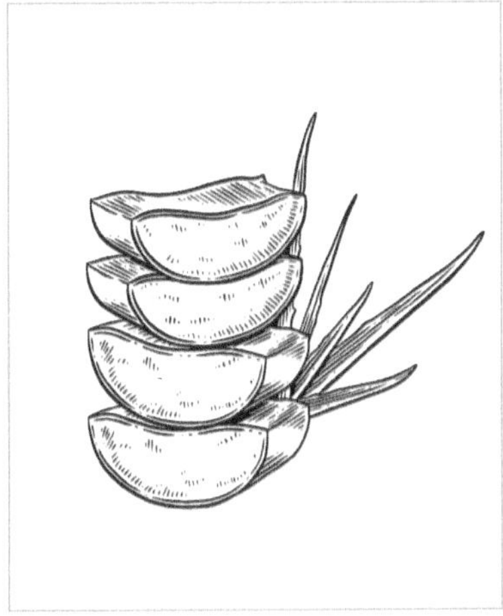

Figure 28

Key Takeaways:

- Probiotics are cultured bacteria that come in food or supplement form.
- Taking a probiotic supplies helpful bacteria to the gut, which helps the gut microbiome come back into balance.
- Probiotics need to be in a high enough dosage to be effective.
- Prebiotics are nutrients that supply probiotic bacteria food and energy and help them thrive.
- Collagen, L-glutamine, and Aloe Vera are supplements that are helpful in supporting gut health.

10

NATURAL SOOTHING REMEDIES FOR DIGESTIVE SYMPTOMS

At this point in the book, you've discovered some positive and impactful changes you can make with your gut health, and perhaps you've already started implementing them. But how can you manage discomfort while you're healing? While all digestive symptoms pose a challenge to living your life, bloating can be especially difficult. To illustrate, my friend Sam shared her experience with me that she went through a few years back.

SAM HAS BEEN LOOKING FORWARD to the pool party this Friday night for weeks now. She's gone shopping to add a cute beach cover-up to her bathing suit ensemble, and everything will be complete after her fingernails and toenails are painted to go perfectly with her skin tone and outfit. It's been a long time since she's been out, and she got a text earlier today confirming that her friend's cute cousin is coming. The last time she saw him at game night, she could tell there was an energy between them as they flirtatiously argued over who had the cleverest card combo in Cards Against Humanity. Truthfully, she's been kicking herself that she didn't suggest they get together for a run at the park later that week. Getting another chance to gauge his interest in her feels exciting, bringing attention to her top priority: feeling as confident as possible in a bathing suit. *Just don't eat anything that will cause you to bloat*, she reminds herself. Sure, no problem—if she could actually figure out what on earth has been causing so much bloating recently. The last three months have been more frustrating than she can express with words. She's been bloated 90 percent of the time, despite cutting out bread and white carbs like that influencer she follows said to do, and she's been on point with her vegetable intake and eating more whole foods than ever. She's been hitting the gym and doing resistance training. It's getting old, real fast. Most of the time, she can't even tell if she's on the right track or gaining weight. Now that it's summer, she's just tired of looking four months pregnant. It's harder to hide her bloating in tank tops and shorts. Baggy T-shirts have been her best friend during this season. *Maybe it's better just to not to eat at all the day of the party*, she thinks. It sounds miserable, but she'd rather deal with a grumbling stomach than risk becoming bloated before hanging around everyone in a bathing suit. But wait, she remembers she tried that before, and it resulted in her getting sick two hours into the party and vomiting in the bathroom from drinking on an empty stomach. Not cute. *Definitely not an option if I want to connect with the guy and leave a good impression*, she thinks. Ruminating between the options gets her feeling anxious, worried, and bummed out. Things probably won't turn out the way she hoped on Friday, anyway. Maybe it's better to show up later after people are done being in the pool or just stay home entirely.

Can you relate at all? Perhaps you've found yourself having a similar internal conversation on particular occasions. Unpredictable and mysterious bloating can turn daily decision-making into a nightmare when you're not sure what's bothering you. What makes this area of digestive health so nebulous is that bloating can be inconsistent, feel random, and impossible to figure out. With the information you now have about SIBO, leaky gut, fiber, and FODMAPS, you'll have more tools to figure this out. But you still could use a few tips, tricks, and strategies to use while you're healing. This chapter will uncover the most important things to know about bloating and steps you can take to do something about it today.

COMMON BLOATING MYTHS

Myth #1 – Bloating Always Means Something Is Wrong

It's normal to bloat after a meal on occasion. When bloating is an everyday issue and takes a long time to go away, that is a sign of imbalances or poor digestion. If you are having frequent bouts of painful bloating, that is potentially a sign of a deeper issue. Experiencing bloat can come from gas, constipation, food you're eating, and medications.

MYTH #2 – Beans Make You Bloat, So Avoid Them

In the last chapter, we discussed lectins and how some people are more sensitive to them. If beans are not pressure-cooked, they have more lectins. This causes more bloating and gas in some individuals, no matter how well you chew. Additionally, if you haven't eaten beans in a while and then reintroduce them, it's possible they will cause bloating. This is normal, since your body isn't used to digesting them and may need an adjustment period. However, not all individuals are sensitive to lectin, so for these individuals, cutting beans from their diet will not improve their bloating and gut health symptoms. When introducing a food you feel will make you have bloating or other symptoms, add a spoonful to start and slowly increase the amount every day over a two-week period. By the end of the two weeks, assess your tolerance of that food as you've slowly increased the amount. Are you experiencing a lot of abdominal discomfort, bloating, and gas around the time of eating this food and afterward? Take note of what you experience.

Myth #3 – Bloating Means You Have a Gluten or Dairy Sensitivity

While gluten and dairy are common culprits for bloating and food intolerance, consumption of them is not always the reason an individual may be experiencing bloating. Going gluten-free has become a popular dietary trend in the past ten years, but only 13 percent of surveyed individuals can claim some form of sensitivity to gluten.[1] While some experts argue that gluten should not be included in our diet at all due to the glue-like action gluten takes on in the body, others warn that cutting it from the diet can cause nutritional deficiencies of fiber, vitamins, minerals. Become an expert on your body through testing and trying out an elimination diet to discover the true answer for yourself.

What's Causing My Bloating?

There is rarely a sole reason you may be bloating. Let's take a look at some reasons for bloating, both common and less common.

Constipation

There's nothing quite as annoying as not being able to have a bowel movement. It's painful, crampy, and it can be frustrating to notice you're bloating after a few days without going. Constipation, or having a bowel movement less than three times per week, happens when stool begins to accumulate and back up in the colon. This causes digested food to stay in your body for a longer period of time. Reasons for this include dehydration, lack of movement, medications, medical conditions, and dietary patterns. There are times when there is no known reason for constipation, and this can be the most frustrating of all. Other classifying symptoms that point to constipation are painful, dry, hard, or lumpy bowel movements and a feeling like you haven't emptied out all the stool.

Before you reach for a laxative, think again. Many people are prescribed a laxative by their doctor to "get things moving." Common brand-name laxatives recommended by physicians are Miralax and Dulcolax. While occasional use of a laxative or stool softener is probably not going to cause you harm, persistent use of laxatives can create dependency in your body. With regular laxative use, the intestines lose muscle and have difficulty with nerve communication. The inside of the intestine widens and is less effective at evacuating stool from the body. The challenge with going to the bathroom makes you need more of the laxative to have a bowel movement.

Ways to Relieve Constipation

- **Don't allow yourself to become dehydrated.** Adults need anywhere from two liters to half their body weight (in pounds) in ounces of water per day. It does vary per person, as the need for hydration is based on temperature, sweating, activity level, and more. If constipation is a regular issue for you, begin keeping track of this and bring a water bottle with you everywhere you go. It's easier to drink more water if you have a one-liter bottle at your desk rather than having to get up multiple times throughout the day to get a glass of water.

- **Get moving.** Exercise stimulates peristalsis, the involuntary, smooth muscle contractions of the intestines. If you're not used to exercising, an easy place to start is walking thirty minutes three times per week, working your way up to five times per week. If you can walk thirty to sixty minutes most days of the week at a moderate to brisk pace, this will support your digestive system as well as your cardiovascular, brain, and metabolic health.

- **Incorporate dietary fiber from fruits, vegetables and legumes.** Insoluble fibers add bulk to your stool, which helps the intestines push it forward and out in a timely manner. However, too much of a good thing is not good. Eating too much fiber—more than forty grams per day—could be a reason for constipation. Supplementing fiber may help some, but it's beneficial to your gut health and the health of each body system if you get this fiber from food you're eating. The best way to do this is to get it from a wide variety of fruits, vegetables, legumes, nuts, seeds, and fermented vegetables. Getting soluble fiber daily from beans can be an additional leg of support in digestive regularity.

- **Take the natural, herbal supplement senna.** Senna is a plant that contains compounds that help with stimulating the nerves in the gut and encourages bowel movements.[2] While it should not be relied on or taken for long periods, it is a better choice for the gut than chemically constructed pharmaceutical medications.

- **Incorporate prebiotic and probiotic foods.** Not only are they highlighted as a way to improve the diversity and health of your gut microbiome, probiotics may help with chronic constipation. When you improve the balance and diversity of your microbial population, this has marvelous alleviating effects on constipation.[3] Prebiotics help probiotics to be even more effective, so you can boost your gut health by getting both. The fibers inside prebiotic foods also help to increase the frequency of bowel movements and soften stool.

- **Take a natural fiber supplement.** Psyllium husk and glucomannan are fibers that can assist with adding bulk to stool so your digestive system can move it along. Glucomannan is a soluble fiber and prebiotic found in the konjac plant, but it can be easily found on the grocery store shelves in shirataki noodles and rice. Psyllium fiber is often seen as "psyllium husk" and originates from the Plantago plant. The fibers come from the seeds or husk of the plant and are often added to packaged cereals. Rich in soluble fibers, psyllium husk acts on the digestive system by pulling water into the colon and softening stool.

- **Give yourself an abdominal massage.** Although this technique is not one you'd expect to relieve constipation, it can make a huge difference. Massaging your abdomen can encourage stool to move along your colon and can reduce cramping and bloating. On the right side of your stomach by your pelvic bone, massage in a circular motion while you move up toward your rib bones. Massage each section for about a minute. Once you reach the rib bone on the right side, take a minute to make your way straight across to the left side of your rib bone. From there, massage downward toward your left pelvic bone and then up to your belly button. You can repeat the circuit for ten minutes, always moving in a clockwise motion.

- **Use the correct positioning for pooping.** The best position for pooping, with or without constipation, is having your knees slightly higher than your hips by using a low step stool to elevate your feet and allowing your abdomen to bulge out slightly.

Excess Gas

Gas production is a natural part of digestion, but excessive gas can be a clue that you've eaten too fast or that something is not right in your digestive tract. Gut bacteria produce gas as they ferment and digest carbohydrates. If carbohydrates and other food components are not digested enough prior to reaching the large intestine, you can experience more gas and bloating. This could be due to poor gut health or food intolerances. Chewing your food well, avoiding excessive water and liquid consumption, and taking probiotics are good first steps to take to alleviate excess gas and bloating. Instead of taking over-the-counter medications like Rolaid and Beano, take activated charcoal tablets. Activated charcoal is a natural binder that can support reduction in bloating and gas. It's great to have on hand, and it really does work.

Water Retention

Strength training, high-intensity workouts, and eating more carbohydrates and salt are all reasons your body may be hanging onto more water and possibly making your feel puffy and bloated. Have you been doing more strength training or intense workouts? It's completely normal for your body to hang onto some water after your muscles have been worked out through strength training, running, and high-intensity workouts. The body holds onto a few grams of water for every gram of glycogen harvested from carbohydrates. Salt is similar in the way that the body holds onto water to maintain proper sodium balance in the body. As the salt is utilized and eliminated, water will be eliminated with it. Packaged, canned, and frozen foods have the most sodium in them. Salt may have an effect on gut bacteria that increases gas.

POOR POSTURE and Positioning

If you lie down right after eating, it takes longer for your body to digest and move the food along your intestinal tract compared to if you are standing. If you're struggling with bloating, taking a quick walk after eating can encourage smooth digestion, reducing gas and bloating.

ANXIETY AND STRESS

With the direct connection between our brain and gut, feelings of anxiousness affect your intestinal tract. Stress contributes to higher levels of the stress hormone cortisol and will impact digestive patterns and result in bloating.

ADDITIONAL WAYS TO **Reduce Bloating**

- **Figure out your food sensitivities through testing and eliminating.** To save yourself from eliminating more foods than you need to, it may be in your best interest to get your blood, skin, and muscles tested prior to doing an elimination diet. You might think it would be redundant to go through three different methods of testing, but this is surprisingly not true. Skin testing can be helpful for environmental allergies such as cat dander, dust mites, and ragweed, but it may not reveal food sensitivities. Food sensitivities are more reliably revealed after blood and muscle testing. After going through both of them myself, I found removing those sensitivities to be much easier. It made more sense to me and became concrete, as I looked at both test results and could confirm with two separate sets of data that I was sensitive to casein, whey, and corn. To my delight, after removing these for six months, I felt the best I ever had.
- **Eat your vegetables cooked rather than raw.** Large, raw salads seem like the poster meal for the healthiest choice in the book, but there are a few reasons why this could be a culprit in causing bloating. First, salads are full of raw, crunchy, and fibrous veggies. Raw vegetables take more effort, time, and enzyme action to

digest and break down, even if you chew them well. This could result in bloating from some of the food particles reaching your colon before being completely broken down, causing the undigested particles to ferment in the colon and release gasses. This can look like bloating, belching, and flatulence. Both are no fun to deal with regularly. Cruciferous vegetables like kale, broccoli, and cabbage are nutrient powerhouses, but they have a strong, fibrous structure and take extra work to break down and digest if eaten raw. Second, most nutrition advice saying to "fill your plate with veggies" and "eat the rainbow" can get us thinking that we must eat large volumes of vegetables no matter who we are and what's going on inside. This is a large volume of food, which will naturally stretch the stomach somewhat as you're digesting that volume down. This is completely normal, but it's still helpful to remember this as a contributing factor. Third, not everyone's digestive system is in the healthiest place. Many people have a poor quality of gut health, leaky gut, and low diversity in their microbiome, meaning they are just not in the same place to digest certain foods as someone with a healthy gut. A healthy digestive tract, enzymes, and microbiome is required to properly break these down and digest them.

- **Avoid or reduce carbonated drinks.** Sparkling water, sodas, or anything carbonated contains bubbles, which can cause abdominal bloating and distention in the intestines after consumption.
- **Reduce added sugars, salt, seed oils, and trans-saturated fats.** The best way to reduce these in your diet is by cooking and baking at home.
- **Consider adding in a digestive enzyme.** Our pancreas and small intestine make enzymes

naturally, but sometimes our body can be deficient. As you heal your gut and reduce inflammation, you'll encourage your organs' ability to produce them. An enzyme supplement can help you as you're healing your gut. A good digestive enzyme supplement contains amylase, lipase, protease, lactase, and sucrase. Like laxatives, avoid taking enzymes consistently for a long period of time so your body doesn't start relying on the external supply and make less of its own.

- **Drink soothing herbal teas.** (You can find specific formulations and recommended dosages in the bonus PDF that comes along with this book.)
- **Peppermint tea** (for nausea, bloating, inflammation) – This tea is known to soothe an upset stomach, nausea, and bloating. It has a relaxing effect on the stomach muscles and calms down inflammation. It's believed to have this effect due to the high concentration of flavonoids, which act to soothe the gut bacteria that give off gases and create bloating. It is also used in homeopathic medicine as a treatment for migraine headaches.
- **Calendula tea** (antiparasitic, detoxifying, helps decrease inflammation) – Calendula is a flower that can be harvested and used to decrease inflammation in the gut wall, [4] aid in detoxifying harmful microbes and substances, and help act against parasitic infections in the body.
- **Ginger tea** (for nausea, bloating, inflammation) – The active compound in ginger is gingerol, which helps gut motility and does not allow food to stay too long in the stomach or intestines. It is an ancient remedy used worldwide, commonly used to treat an upset stomach. Ginger also contains antioxidant and anti-

inflammatory properties. It's even been used to treat pain due to this effect.

- **Chamomile tea** (for upset stomach, bloating, anxiety, restless sleep) – Chamomile helps balance out harmful and helpful gut microbes and soothe the digestive system. It has both anti-inflammatory and antimicrobial properties. Chamomile has even been used as a natural supplement for treating acne, eczema, and rosacea.
- **Fennel tea** (for constipation, bloating, gas, abdominal pain) – Fennel in food or tea benefits heart health, digestive health, and healthy weight management because it possesses an array of micronutrients. This herb tastes similar to licorice and has vitamin C, potassium, folate, and fibers that help support various functions inside the body and act as a homeostatic aid.
- **Milk thistle** (for supporting natural liver detoxification and bile flow) – Inside milk thistle is a flavonoid called silymarin, which is believed to help relieve any toxin burdens from the liver. It's usually suggested to people with liver inflammation.[5]
- **Nettle** (for natural anti-inflammatory support) – Known for its anti-inflammatory and antioxidant properties, nettle has been used to decrease inflammation in prostate conditions and is now being studied as a potential therapy for obesity, insulin resistance, and digestive health.[6]
- **Turmeric** (anti-inflammatory) – Turmeric (curcumin) is a brightly colored orange root that has been used around the world for its anti-inflammatory, blood-sugar supporting, and pain-relieving properties. It can help in healing the gut after taking a course of antibiotics, and it helps balance the gut flora as well. It may help decrease chances of developing stomach

ulcers and infections, such as gastritis, due to how it helps balance gut mucosa. Additionally, turmeric may be helpful in neutralizing unhelpful bacteria in the gut and help heal the gut lining.[7]

<u>KEY TAKEAWAYS:</u>

- To help relieve digestive discomfort and bloating, lean toward steamed or cooked vegetables instead of eating large amounts of raw vegetables.
- Incorporating herbal remedies and teas can be helpful in supporting your digestive symptoms as you heal your gut.

11

WHAT IT TAKES TO MAKE WEIGHT LOSS SUSTAINABLE: A GUT-HEALTH CENTERED APPROACH

Remember in the beginning of this book when I shared about my troubling skin rash and steady weight gain? While initiating a gut healing protocol and lifestyle was a huge part of the solution, it was far from my first attempt to fix how I looked and felt.

Several years prior, in 2015, a woman reached out to me and invited me to join her team that sells diet and exercise programs. Desperate to lose weight and feel more confident about my body, I decided to join her. I began selling an exercise and weight loss program that intended to simplify foods and came with a nutrient-dense shake. While I enjoyed the intention and the idea of discipline, I realized that, with the shake, there were two tiny servings of fat and two small servings of carbohydrates you were allowed each day. Here I was, previously eating cereal, sandwiches, pasta, and desserts. This shift was so drastic for my brain and body that I started getting intense cravings for the foods I wanted. I didn't have the discernment at the time to avoid extreme diet and exercise programs, and I frequently gave into cravings and disordered eating behaviors. This experience was a huge detour that rerouted me from recovering from disordered eating. When I reflect on that time, I saw how other people in my online community swore by eating this way and working out at such a high intensity for months at a time. I recall how frustrated I felt that my results never seemed to arrive, and I instead backslid in my relationship with food and into vicious binge-eating and purging cycles that took weeks to bounce back from.

The misconception most people make with extreme programs is that you can do the program with discipline alone. If you give into cravings, you feel like a failure and decide you must be mentally weak and lack self-control. Weight loss attempts with crash dieting, drastically cutting calories and food groups, puts your body in stress response. Within twelve to twenty-four hours, our body uses up the glycogen energy stores in the liver and muscles as it senses energy intake is more minor, preparing for starvation mode. The next two days, as this stress continues, cortisol is released into the bloodstream at higher levels, causing the body to retain more water, increasing bloating. At this point, the body slows down the metabolism to make up for what it perceives as food scarcity or starvation. At three days, your body prefers to store more fat for energy and begins breaking down lean muscle because it senses starvation. As we've reviewed throughout this book, the excess stress will affect the gut, creating a higher chance for leaky gut and unhealthy bacteria to populate. Drastically reducing your calories for prolonged periods may also cause nutrient deficiencies, which is a recipe for disaster with your gut health.

Meanwhile, your metabolic rate slows way down, and this reduces your thyroid and adrenaline production. This reduction creates a feeling of exhaustion, and you feel a general lack of physical and mental energy. At one week, much of your weight loss has been from lean muscle mass. If the restriction is continued, the appetite-stimulating hormone ghrelin builds up in your system, which makes it much easier to binge eat. Your mood will suffer, and your thoughts will be constantly preoccupied with food.

Once you decide to stop dieting, most likely you begin eating the foods that were off-limits while on your diet, and your body begins to store fat to replenish energy stores. The fat cells of our body remember the earlier starvation, and the original level of body fat can be reached more quickly after an extreme diet. Often, the amount of fat increases more than before.[1]

If crash diets aren't working for us, what can be done instead? If your goal is to lose weight, the right mentality requires you to view your goal as a long game. When you crash diet, the focus isn't about learning how to be healthy and live life as the person you want to become. Instead, you get distracted by reaching your goal as quickly as possible, with the illusion that you'll be happy once you reach your goal. This isn't true, and any program or solution selling this as a result is being dishonest and promoting short-term thinking. We've been sold the short-term-thinking, fast-results lie for far too long, and we're not buying it anymore. Deep down, we know what we really need is a shift from short-term thinking to long-term thinking. When you succeed at reframing your weight loss efforts into a long-term-thinking approach, you find that the strategy you commit yourself to is sustainable, mindful, and a slow burn in the direction of your goal. Getting away from the "all or nothing" or "on and off the wagon" mentality will do more for you than reduce your body fat and explode your confidence; you will also extinguish that smoldering fire of inflammation and stress within. You'll have the opportunity to gradually implement strategies at a pace that works for you, allowing you to sustainably release weight while keeping a healthy gut and good hormone levels. My sole desire is that you see through false marketing strategies from businesspeople and companies looking to make a quick buck off of you as a consumer who deeply wants to change your life and from there come into agreement with healthy lifestyle involving the power of long-term thinking that will get you sticky results. What if you could reach a place where you don't gain back the weight you lost and then some? That's the goal, isn't it? It becomes helpful to look at it this way: Which of the two options below would you choose?

- Getting the results you want in eight weeks, but then realizing how difficult it is to keep up the diet and workout schedule at this level of intensity. You decide to stop and take a break, but you find you don't want to restart the plan you're on. You become discouraged and slide back into worse habits than before, decreasing your overall health.
- Getting the results you want in two to six months, but having your body adapt to the change at a realistic pace, so the positive changes you've made become part of your routine and feel effortless to maintain. The positive changes you've made to your lifestyle improve your gut health, metabolic health, immune system, and heart health.

I DON'T KNOW about you, but the second option sounds much more sustainable in the long-term. I know I would be much less likely to slip back into unhealthy habits like crash dieting or restricting food even if I felt uncomfortable about my weight or how clothes were fitting. My brain, fully functioning and not undernourished, would be much more likely to become aware of this, be equipped to make better decisions, make a slight course correction, and keep going.

Even if your goal is not to lose weight, adopting long-term thinking will always give you better answers, solutions, and results in everything you set out to do.

Now, for the news I've been building up to all along. What is the key to effectively losing weight while keeping your health? Following these steps below in combination with each other.

THE GUT-HEALTHY WAY TO **Lose Weight**

- **Incorporate the knowledge from this book about stress management, medications, and food.** When you build your lifestyle around gut health as a priority, you reduce inflammation, improve nutrient absorption, become happier and more energetic, and weight loss becomes easier.
- **Switch from shakes, bars, and processed freezer meals** to home-cooked, minimal-ingredient, whole-food meals 95 percent of the time.
- **Engage in strength training three to six days per week for 30 minutes or more.** Stop doing only cardio and high-intensity exercise with light weights. Add weight lifting or training with resistance bands and do brisk walking most days. Try to time your meals to be thirty minutes before the start of a workout. Strength training builds muscle tone and strength, which helps protect you from injury and improves your metabolism and ability to process carbohydrates and sugar. Growing and maintaining muscles also helps fire up the metabolism as it burns more energy.
- **Swap your sugar for nonglycemic sweeteners** such as monk fruit and allulose.

- **Ensure you're sleeping eight to nine hours each night.**
- **Keep stress levels in check** with the strategies such as diaphragmatic breathing.
- **Eat grass-fed organ meats.** Beef organs such as liver, heart, and brain have rich vitamin profiles that are readily bioavailable for our body to use and heal what's damaged. They help support hormone production while you're in a caloric deficit.
- **Use a gentle caloric deficit when losing fat.** As your body heals from the inside out, it will need to be in a caloric deficit to burn fat (think 200 to 250 calories). Make sure you're strength training to stimulate muscle growth so your body is burning the fat and not muscle.
- **Eat adequate protein.** Consume 0.75-1g/lb of protein of your goal weight. For example, if your goal weight is 130 pounds and you weigh 150 pounds, consume 97-130 grams of protein daily.

MOST OF MY weight loss happened naturally when I finally began eating enough of the right food. Notice how I didn't say you needed a shake or to drink half your weight in water to do this? Since weight loss can be inhibited by inflammation and poor gut and adrenal health, many people find that even a strict caloric deficit can't help them. This is called weight loss resistance and can absolutely be reversed by the steps I mentioned and a bit of patience. Focusing on supporting my gut health allowed me to unlock everything I had ever wanted in my health.

Cut ties with the old way and step into the long-term focused way of living—you'll thank me later! As you come to the end of this book, you face a new, bright beginning. The Four-Week Gut Health Reset Plan is outlined after the conclusion, and I've written this plan carefully with you in mind. I thought of challenges you might currently be facing as you read this and how you could troubleshoot them with ease. I considered the timeline and how I could help you incorporate health-minded habits at a realistic pace. The truth of the matter is that you're going to want to continue healing your gut past the four weeks, so I've included a guide to help you all the way to six months and beyond.

KEY TAKEAWAY:

- Focusing on your gut health as a priority will help make fat loss easier and more sustainable.

CONCLUSION

I've always believed that if gut health and nutrition could be explained in an approachable way and made a little less intimidating, more people would jump at the opportunity to do more for their gut microbiome — without delay! The steps to improving your gut health are simple but not always straightforward when integrating them into your life. Remember, don't view this as a race...view this as a marathon. If I could give you any parting words, it would be don't wait to start the gut healing plan. Work on switching over to whole-foods cooking, moving more, and improving sleep in a gradual progression, adding one or two things in until you've got the hang of it, so you don't overwhelm yourself and give up. If you feel like you need additional support, working with a gut health coach and nutritionist or partnering with a holistic doctor could be life changing. I'd be happy to support you at my practice or help point you in the right direction, so don't hesitate to reach out. Thinking about you reading this book from cover to cover fills me with excitement and anticipation for what you're about to uncover. I pray that what's written in these pages changes your life even more than it changed mine. When you heal your gut, the rest will follow!

YOUR FOUR-WEEK GUT HEALTH RESET PLAN

You can also download a free color copy of this plan with progress tracking worksheets in the bonus PDF that comes with your purchase of this book.

Before you get started, here are some suggestions I know you will find helpful in the long-term:

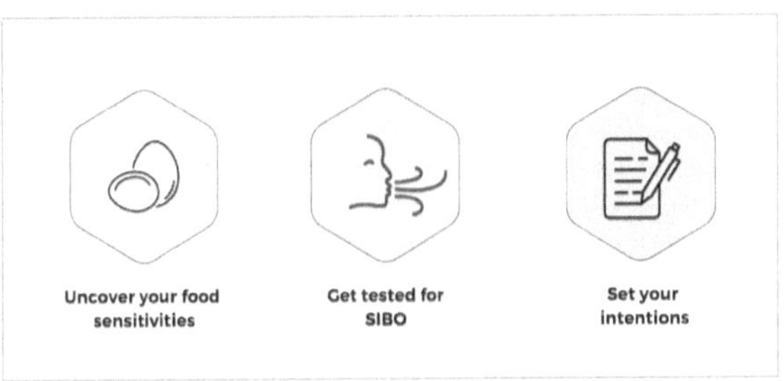

Figure 29

- Learn which foods you're sensitive to and form a plan
- Take a breath test to discover if you have SIBO/SIFO. You'll want to take herbal antimicrobials in addition to probiotics if SIBO/SIFO is present. In general, natural herbs are safe to take, so if you have you have all the

symptoms you could still go ahead and do the plan with the SIBO recommendations after getting your doctor's approval. Breath testing device recommendations are in the back of this book.

- Set your intentions for the next four weeks and what you want your health to look like from here on out. Knowing what you want as an end result can help with moral when things get challenging.

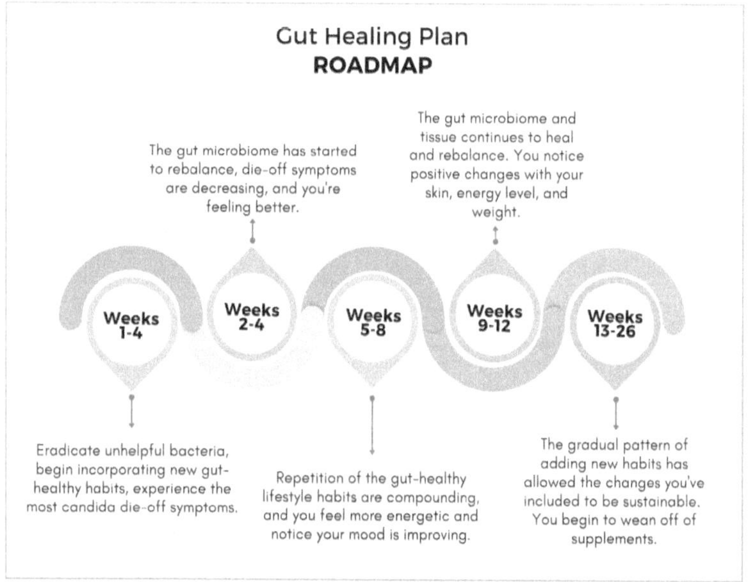

Figure 30

Forming Gut-Healthy Habits

During the first four weeks of your gut-healing journey, the lifestyle and nutrition habits in figure 31 will make the biggest difference at the beginning. The remaining habits found in figure 36 can be added in at any time. It's normal to feel like you need to change everything as soon as possible, but remember to apply long-term thinking and go at a pace that is realistic for you. Your lifestyle around sleep, movement, and nutrition has the biggest impact on your gut health, and the status of your gut will influence how strong your immune system and metabolic health will be. Supplements are meant to be an addition to a set of healthy habits, and your goal should never be to just add supplements to the mix without changing any of your habits. That's when it starts to look like throwing money directly in the trash. You cheat yourself, and you don't make the progress you could by setting the foundation with habits.

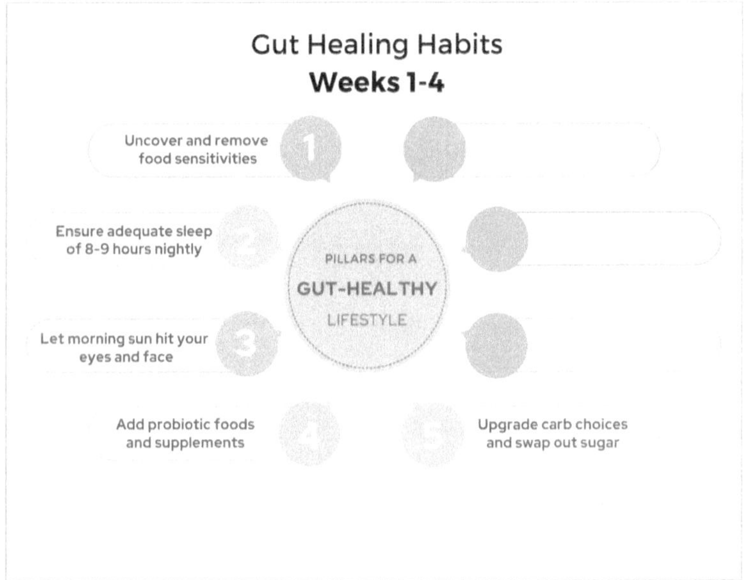

Figure 31

When looking at the Gut Healing Plan, you'll notice the mention of a morning detox elixir and a supplement called Triplex. The elixir is a prebiotic and probiotic drink that may support a reduction in candida, improve digestion, stabilize blood sugar, and encourage the development of a healthy gut microbiome.[1] Lemons provide vitamin C and prebiotic fibers, and apple cider vinegar is a fermented apple juice drink that has probiotic qualities. Triplex is prebiotic supplement that aids in blood sugar balance and weight loss. Gut dysbiosis, insulin resistance and elevated fasting blood sugar are often seen together, and each one can contribute to weight loss resistance. Triplex will be most helpful to those who are looking for an extra leg of support with appetite balance, fat loss, and improving their blood sugar and insulin levels while healing their gut. More information can be found in the Resources section of this book.

4-WEEK PLAN 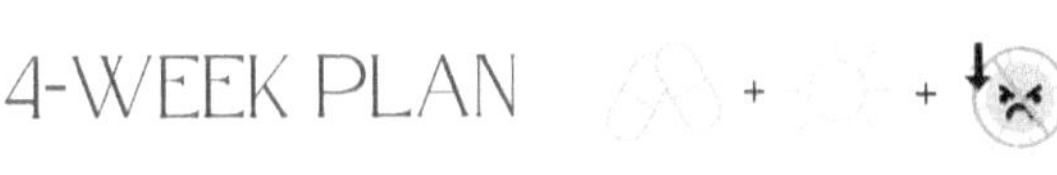

PHASE 1

Goal: Reduce Harmful Bacteria, Lower Inflammation, Begin Gut-Healing Habits, and Manage Symptoms

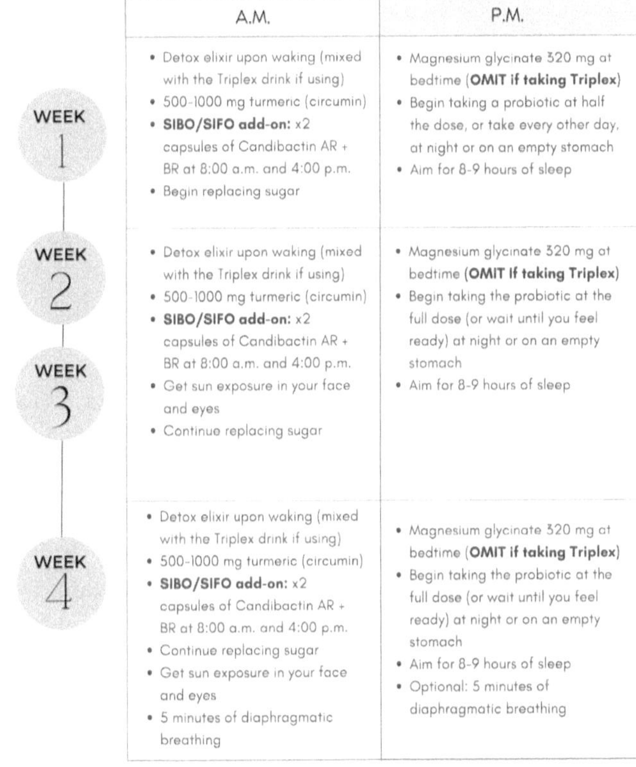

	A.M.	P.M.
WEEK 1	• Detox elixir upon waking (mixed with the Triplex drink if using) • 500-1000 mg turmeric (circumin) • **SIBO/SIFO add-on:** x2 capsules of Candibactin AR + BR at 8:00 a.m. and 4:00 p.m. • Begin replacing sugar	• Magnesium glycinate 320 mg at bedtime (**OMIT if taking Triplex**) • Begin taking a probiotic at half the dose, or take every other day, at night or on an empty stomach • Aim for 8-9 hours of sleep
WEEK 2 **WEEK 3**	• Detox elixir upon waking (mixed with the Triplex drink if using) • 500-1000 mg turmeric (circumin) • **SIBO/SIFO add-on:** x2 capsules of Candibactin AR + BR at 8:00 a.m. and 4:00 p.m. • Get sun exposure in your face and eyes • Continue replacing sugar	• Magnesium glycinate 320 mg at bedtime (**OMIT if taking Triplex**) • Begin taking the probiotic at the full dose (or wait until you feel ready) at night or on an empty stomach • Aim for 8-9 hours of sleep
WEEK 4	• Detox elixir upon waking (mixed with the Triplex drink if using) • 500-1000 mg turmeric (circumin) • **SIBO/SIFO add-on:** x2 capsules of Candibactin AR + BR at 8:00 a.m. and 4:00 p.m. • Continue replacing sugar • Get sun exposure in your face and eyes • 5 minutes of diaphragmatic breathing	• Magnesium glycinate 320 mg at bedtime (**OMIT if taking Triplex**) • Begin taking the probiotic at the full dose (or wait until you feel ready) at night or on an empty stomach • Aim for 8-9 hours of sleep • Optional: 5 minutes of diaphragmatic breathing

Download the bonus PDF guide for Weeks 5 and beyond.

Figure 32

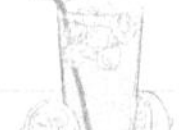

Figure 33

Helpful Tips for Phase 1

- The first four weeks are likely going to be the most
  challenging in terms of symptoms. This is because as
  bad microorganisms die off, they release endotoxins,
  which can result in you feeling some things. Bloating,
  diarrhea, constipation, gas, body aches, headaches,
  joint pain, fatigue or low energy, tiredness, and
  changes in sleep and appetite are not uncommon
  during the die-off period. This usually gets better in
  two weeks or less, but some people report symptoms
  up to two months. Magnesium is also helpful in
  supporting natural detoxification pathways, which is
  why it's included as a supplement in Phase 1.
- Rather than eating lots of raw vegetables, try cooking
  most of them for easier digestion. Follow food eating

techniques from the previous chapters by avoiding snacking and allowing three to five hours between meals, walking after eating, and chewing adequately. This will support healthy gut motility, balanced microbes, and regulation of bowel movements.

- If you're able, take a high-quality omega-3 supplement such as Nordic Naturals to support anti-inflammatory action in the body and brain health.
- Add in a collagen supplement. Taking twenty grams of collagen daily can support reduction in bloating and digestive symptoms.[2] Collagen powder, bone broth protein, and regular bone broth are excellent sources of collagen, protein, and essential minerals.
- Work toward switching any store-bought, sugary baked goods with your own homemade baked goods. There are over one hundred gut-friendly recipes on my social media accounts, so I encourage you to check those out.
- Another helpful strategy during Phase 1 for many will be to reduce FODMAP foods and carbohydrates to support reduction in yeast and unhealthy microbes. Eat whole foods and reduce processed, packaged foods as much as you can.
- Incorporate probiotic foods during Phase 1 to support rebalancing of the gut microbiome.
- A quality digestive enzyme can help here as well if you're having a lot of bloating or symptoms after eating. I recommend Standard Process Enzycore, as it has a combination of all the pancreatic digestive enzymes. You can look it up online or read more about where I get mine in the bonus PDF.
- When taking turmeric, you can choose either powder or capsule form. Choosing a supplement with berberine can help support a decrease in inflammation, improve liver detoxification and lower

internal stress, assisting with weight loss and gut healing.[3]

- For positive SIBO / SIFO, take two capsules of Candibactin AR + BR twice per day for four weeks. These are strong herbal supplements designed to eradicate bad microbes from the gut. This exact regimen was just as effective, if not more so, than antibiotic treatment with Rifaximin.[4]

A Week of Gut-Healthy Eating

Eating for a healthy gut focuses around eating real, whole food and reducing the burden that inflammatory food additives, trans-saturated fats, added sugars, and preservatives put on our digestive system. The meals and recipes included in this section are mostly gluten-free, dairy-free, and sugar-free. Here is an example of what eating for gut health could look like:

Day 1

- **Breakfast:** Veggie egg scramble
- **Lunch:** Taco bowls
- **Dinner:** Seared salmon with mashed cauliflower
- **Snack or Dessert:** Grain-free chocolate chip cookies

Day 2

- **Breakfast:** Protein waffle with monk fruit maple syrup, nut butter, and berries
- **Lunch:** Superfood salad
- **Dinner:** Chicken meatloaf skillet with spaghetti squash
- **Snack or Dessert:** 80 percent or above monk-fruit sweetened dark chocolate and nut butter

Day 3

- **Breakfast:** Old-fashioned oats and coconut yogurt bowl with berries, hemp seeds, chia seeds, and nut butter
- **Lunch:** Mediterranean chicken salad
- **Dinner:** Cheesy butternut squash bowl
- **Snack or Dessert:** Chocolate zucchini bread

Day 4

- **Breakfast:** High-protein chocolate breakfast cake topped with berries
- **Lunch:** Salmon teriyaki bowl
- **Dinner:** Roasted red pepper soup
- **Snack or Dessert:** Healthy banana pudding

Day 5

- **Breakfast:** Blueberry maple overnight oats
- **Lunch:** Steak and veggie fajita bowl
- **Dinner:** Mushroom protein bowl
- **Snack or Dessert:** Blueberry cardamom muffins

Day 6

- **Breakfast:** Triple berry collagen smoothie
- **Lunch:** Curry chicken salad
- **Dinner:** Turkey burgers with sweet potato fries
- **Snack or Dessert:** Almond butter cups

Day 7

- **Breakfast:** Zucchini, onion, and pepper scramble and blueberries
- **Lunch:** Grass-fed ground beef quinoa bowl
- **Dinner:** Almond flour crust pizza
- **Snack or Dessert:** Healthy chocolate pudding

Gut-Healthy Grocery List

Vegetables

- Artichoke
- Spinach
- Arugula
- Asparagus
- Broccoli
- Broccoli sprouts
- Brussels sprouts
- Cabbage
- Cauliflower
- Celery
- Cucumber
- Mushrooms
- Radish
- Zucchini
- Beets
- Carrots
- Parsnips
- Pumpkin
- Squash
- Sweet potatoes
- Turnips
- Yams
- Onion

Fruits

- Avocados
- Oranges
- Cherries
- Strawberries
- Tomatoes
- Unsweetened coconut
- Bananas
- Watermelon
- Lemons
- Limes
- Blueberries
- Raspberries
- Blackberries

Nuts & Seeds

- Hemp seeds
- Brazil nuts
- Almonds
- Hazelnuts
- Pumpkin seeds
- Chia seeds
- Pecans
- Walnuts
- Pistachios

Plant-Based Milk

- Almond milk
- Hemp milk
- Coconut milk
- Coconut cream

Fats & Oils

- Avocado oil
- Coconut oil
- Grass-fed ghee
- Grass-fed butter
- Beef tallow
- Duck fat
- Macadamia nut oil
- Olives
- Organic Olive oil
- Almond butter
- Walnut butter
- Coconut butter
- 70-100% Dark chocolate

Legumes & Grains

- Organic Brown rice
- Organic Chickpeas
- Organic Lentils
- Organic Black beans
- Organic Pinto beans
- Organic Quinoa

Proteins

- Organic ground turkey
- Organic, free-range, ground chicken
- Organic 100% grass-fed ground beef
- Anchovies
- Ground lamb
- Mackerel
- Atlantic cod
- Organic bone broth
- Pasture-raised eggs
- Wild-caught salmon
- Organic, free-range chicken
- Collagen powder
- Bone broth protein powder
- Grass-fed beef organs

Herbs & Spices

- Cinnamon
- Cilantro
- Black pepper
- Mint
- Ginger
- Garlic

Figure 34

Herbs & Spices
- Sea salt
- Cloves
- Turmeric

Probiotic foods
- Coconut yogurt
- Sauerkraut
- Kimchi
- Natto
- Refrigerator pickles
- Raw parmesan cheese
- Raw kefir
- Raw grass-fed cheddar
- Kombucha
- Apple cider vinegar

Breads & Flours
- Artisan sourdough bread
- Almond flour
- Coconut flour
- Arrowroot flour

Sweeteners
- Allulose
- Monk fruit extract

Dairy
- Feta cheese
- Raw, grass-fed cheddar
- Raw Parmesan cheese
- 2%-5% Organic Greek Yogurt
- Kefir
- Goat cheese
- Raw sheep's milk cheese

Drinks & Tea
- Filtered water
- Organic coffee
- Matcha green tea
- Dandelion tea
- DGL licorice root tea
- Ginger root
- Ginger tea
- Marshmallow root tea
- Peppermint tea

Figure 35

What to Do After Week 4

- Stop using turmeric, but continue the other supplements.
- Download the free bonus PDF for the next steps to secure the success of your gut-healing journey. It includes your roadmap to building sustainable gut health with more guidance on Phase 1, along with habit trackers, shopping lists, worksheets, and more recipes to make creating new habits easier. You can

also find Phase 2, which you can use to help lay out the next six months of your healing journey.

- Begin increasing diversity of plant-based foods and bring prebiotic fibers in. Aim for twenty to thirty plant-based foods per week, as this supports the highest diversity in gut bacteria.[5]
- Challenge yourself to add a new gut-healthy habit each week to further support your healing. The rest of the habits are revealed in figure 36.

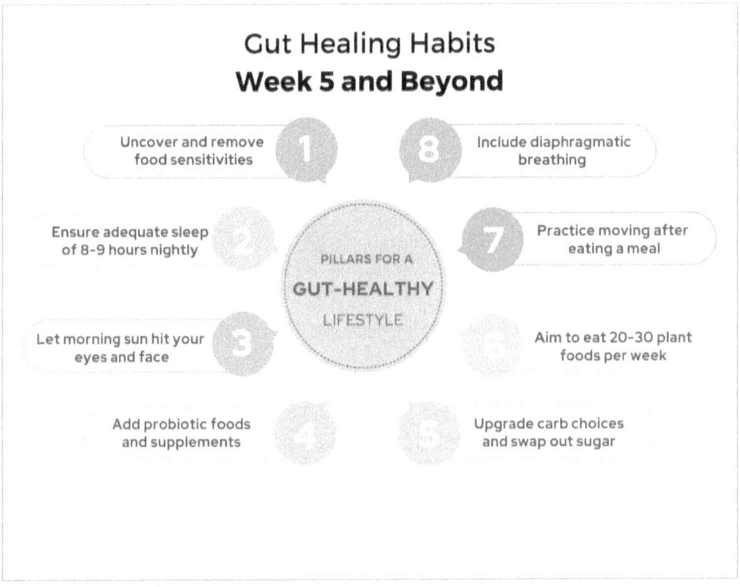

Figure 36

GUT-HEALING RECIPES

Most of the recipes in this section of the book are gluten, dairy, and refined-sugar free. When purchasing foods and condiments, always check the labels to ensure products are free of allergens.

~

BREAKFAST RECIPES

THICK TRIPLE BERRY COLLAGEN SMOOTHIE

Ingredients:

- 1 cup mixed berries (strawberries, blueberries, raspberries)
- 1 cup ice*
- 20 grams of collagen powder**
- 1 tablespoon nut or seed butter
- 1/2 frozen banana***
- 1/3 cup unsweetened nut milk

Instructions:

1. Add all ingredients to a high-speed blender (such as a Vitamix) and turn it on to medium speed. Use a tamper to push the contents into the blades to make a thick smoothie. Keep blending on medium speed for a minute and repeating the process until all ingredients have incorporated into a smooth, consistent texture.

2. Scrape the contents out of the blender into a bowl or glass. Sprinkle toppings onto the surface and enjoy!

*Option: Freeze full-fat coconut milk from a can in an ice cube tray. Do this ahead of time so you can try using a few as part of the ice portion. I like to use 2 frozen coconut milk ice cubes and the rest regular ice. This creates a nice, creamy smoothie.

**Vanilla-flavored collagen from Bulletproof works great here.

***Try to freeze bananas when they're green for better blood sugar balance.

Gut-Healthy, Oil-Free Granola

(Yields approximately 4 cups of granola)

Ingredients:

- 2 cups rolled oats
- 1/2 cup natural almond butter
- 1 tablespoon chia seeds
- 2 tablespoons pumpkin seeds
- 1 banana, mashed
- ¼ cup monk fruit brown sugar
- 1 teaspoon vanilla extract
- ½ teaspoon almond extract
- ¼ teaspoon Ceylon cinnamon

Instructions:

1. Turn the oven on to 350 degrees F. Line a large baking tray with parchment paper and set aside. Mash the banana in a large mixing bowl and stir in the almond butter and monk fruit sweetener. Stir in the remaining ingredients and mix well.

2. Spread the granola onto the baking sheet and press down evenly and no thicker than ½ an inch. Bake for 20-25 minutes until golden brown, tossing it half-way through.

SINGLE-SERVE, HIGH-PROTEIN PUMPKIN WAFFLE

Ingredients:

- 1 large egg
- 2 egg whites
- 3 tablespoons 100% pumpkin purée*
- 1 scoop vanilla protein powder or 1 serving of vanilla collagen
- 1/4 cup rolled oats
- 2 tablespoons almond flour
- 2 teaspoons coconut flour
- 2 teaspoons arrowroot flour
- 1 teaspoon baking powder
- 2 tablespoons granulated allulose
- 1 teaspoon pumpkin pie spice**
- 1 teaspoon coconut oil
- 1 teaspoon almond extract

Instructions:

1. Preheat a waffle iron. Add all wet ingredients to a blender followed by the dry ones. Blend until just incorporated without over-mixing.

2. Using a heat-proof cooking brush, spread some coconut oil on each surface of the waffle iron top and bottom. Cook for about 4-6 minutes, or until the until the indicator light goes off. Serve with sunflower seeds, monk fruit maple syrup, almond butter, and blueberries!

*Omit pumpkin puree and pumpkin pie spice for a standard waffle.

**Make your own pumpkin pie spice with 1/2 teaspoon of cinnamon, 1/4 teaspoon ginger, 1/4 teaspoon cardamom, a pinch of nutmeg, and a pinch of allspice).

Veggie Egg Skillet

(Makes 3-4 servings)

Ingredients:

- 10 large, organic and pasture-raised eggs
- 1/4 cup shredded goat cheese
- 1/3 cup sun-dried tomatoes
- 2 handfuls spinach
- ½ sweet yellow onion, diced
- 1 green pepper, diced
- Sea salt and black pepper to taste
- 1/2 teaspoon garlic powder
- 1-2 tbsp grass-fed butter for cooking

Instructions:

1. Preheat a 12 inch large cast-iron skillet to medium heat. Melt butter in the skillet, then the onion.

2. Sauté the onion for 3 minutes, then add the green pepper and garlic powder and cook another 3 minutes.

3. Beat eggs lightly in a large mixing bowl and mix in the salt and pepper. Add the egg mixture to the skillet. Cook until half the egg mixture is solidified, then add the remaining ingredients. Cook until eggs are completely solid, but fluffy.

Blueberry Maple Protein Overnight "Oats"

(Makes 1 serving)

Ingredients:

- 2 tablespoons hemp seeds
- 2 teaspoons chia seeds
- 1 tablespoon flaxseeds
- 1 tablespoon unsweetened, shredded coconut
- 2 tablespoons coconut yogurt
- ½ serving vanilla bone broth protein powder
- 1 teaspoon vanilla extract
- ½ teaspoon cinnamon
- 1/2 cup unsweetened nut milk
- 2 tablespoons monk fruit maple syrup

Instructions:

1. Combine all ingredients except for blueberries in a jar or glass container. Shake or mix well. Cover and let sit in the fridge for at least 6 hours. Top with blueberries and enjoy.

Chocolate Breakfast Cake with Berries

(Makes 2 servings)

Ingredients:

- 1/4 cup almond flour
- 2 tablespoons coconut flour
- 2 scoops chocolate bone broth protein powder
- 2 tablespoons allulose
- 3 tablespoons cacao powder
- 1 teaspoon baking powder
- 2 tablespoons chia seeds
- 2 tablespoons certified gluten-free steel cut oats
- 2 pasture-raised, organic eggs
- 2 tablespoons coconut yogurt
- 2 tablespoons unsweetened nut milk

Instructions:

1. Preheat oven to 350F. Line a 8x4 baking pan with parchment. You can use an 8x8 pan, just start checking for doneness at 15 min mark.

2. Combine all dry ingredients together in a medium-sized bowl. Add wet ingredients in and mix until smooth with a spatula.

3. Pour into prepped baking dish and bake for 25-30 min, removing from oven when a toothpick comes out clean. Let cool slightly and enjoy. Topping suggestions: nuts, seeds, berries, pears, apple, banana, nut or seed butter.

ZUCCHINI, ONION, AND BELL PEPPER SCRAMBLE

(Makes 2 servings)

Ingredients:

- 1 teaspoon avocado oil
- 6 large organic, pasture-raised eggs
- Sea salt
- Black pepper
- Garlic powder
- 1 medium zucchini, diced
- ½ medium sweet onion, diced
- 1 large green or red bell pepper, diced

Instructions:

1. Prepare vegetables and set aside. Combine eggs and seasonings in a medium mixing bowl and beat with a fork to scramble them.

2. Heat the oil in a large, preheated cast-iron skillet. Add the onions to the skillet and saute for 3-4 minutes until slightly translucent. Add the zucchini and bell pepper and saute another 3-4 minutes. Pour in the egg mixture. Stir frequently until cooked thoroughly.

Lunch and Dinner Recipes

SUPERFOOD PROTEIN SALAD

(makes 2-3 servings)

Ingredients:

- 1 pound organic, pasture-raised chicken breast
- 1 teaspoon garlic powder
- Sea salt and black pepper to taste
- 6 cups of spinach or dark salad greens
- ½ cup fresh blueberries
- ½ cucumber, sliced
- 2 cups broccoli, stemmed and chopped
- ½ medium avocado, sliced
- 2 tablespoons pumpkin seeds
- ¼ cup dairy-free, gut-friendly ranch dressing*
- Optional: Shelled hemp seeds for topping

Instructions:

1. Preheat the oven to 425 degrees F. Prepare a baking sheet with parchment paper. Season the chicken with garlic powder, salt and pepper. Bake for 15-18 minutes, flipping halfway through. Remove from the oven when the internal temperature of the chicken reaches 160 degrees F.

2. While the chicken is baking, steam the broccoli in a medium pot with an inch of water in the base. Turn the heat to medium high and cook until the broccoli is fork-tender.

3. While chicken and broccoli are cooking, place salad greens, cucumber, blueberries, avocado, and pumpkin seeds in a large

mixing bowl. Dice the chicken into bite-sized pieces when done baking and slightly cooled and add to the mixing bowl along with the broccoli. Pour the ranch over the surface and toss with tongs.

*Primal Kitchen makes a ranch dressing free from inflammatory ingredients. You can make your own with just a few simple ingredients. The recipe is included in the bonus PDF guide.

HEALTHY CHICKEN MEATLOAF SKILLET AND SPAGHETTI SQUASH

(Makes 4 servings)

Ingredients:

- 1 organic spaghetti squash, halved and insides discarded
- 2 tablespoons certified organic, cold-pressed olive oil
- 2 cloves garlic, minced
- 1/2 yellow onion, diced
- ½ cup butternut squash, grated
- 1 pound organic, pasture-raised ground chicken
- 1 teaspoon sea salt
- 1/2 teaspoon freshly ground black pepper
- 1/2 teaspoon dried basil
- 1/2 teaspoon dried oregano
- 1/4 cup blanched almond flour
- 1 large, pasture-raised egg
- 1/3 cup low-sugar marinara sauce**
- 1 cup canned marinara sauce
- *Optional:* freshly grated raw parmesan cheese

Instructions:

1. Preheat the oven to 400 degrees F. Prepare a baking sheet with parchment paper. Drizzle ½ tablespoon of olive oil on each inner half of the spaghetti squash and sprinkle with salt and pepper. Place the halves cut side down and poke several holes in the skin with a fork. Bake for 40-50 minutes.

2. While the squash is baking in the oven, heat a medium-sized 10-inch cast-iron skillet to medium heat, then add olive oil. Add the minced garlic and saute for around 30-60 seconds and fragrant. Add the onion and saute for 3 minutes. Add the green

pepper and saute another 3 minutes. Add the ground chicken, butternut squash, and seasonings and stir to combine. Let cook for 4-5 minutes, stirring every so often.

3. Take the chicken and vegetable saute mixture off of heat before it's fully cooked. With the back of a spatula, press the mixture down firmly so the surface is smooth. Pour off any excess liquid if you prefer the end product to be firmer. Spread the marinara sauce evenly over the surface. Place in the 400 degree F preheated oven and bake uncovered for 15-20 minutes. If you have another rack to place it on inside the oven, you can bake both squash and the chicken at the same time. If you don't, wait until the squash is finished baking and then place in the oven.

4. When spaghetti squash is finished baking, let cool slightly. Take a fork and scrape the inside of each squash out into a separate dish. Place spaghetti squash on plates and top with meatloaf skillet. Top with freshly grated raw parmesan cheese if desired.

~

Taco Bowls

(Makes 2-3 servings)

Ingredients:

- 1 tablespoon chili powder
- 1 ½ teaspoons cumin
- 1 teaspoon sea salt
- 1 teaspoon ground black pepper
- ½ teaspoon paprika
- ¼ teaspoon garlic powder
- ¼ teaspoon onion powder
- ¼ teaspoon red pepper flakes
- ¼ teaspoon dried oregano
- 1-pound grass-fed ground beef
- 2 teaspoons avocado or olive oil
- 1 can of black beans (Eden Foods), drained and rinsed*
- 1 tomato, chopped
- ¼ cup white onion, chopped
- 6 cups salad greens (spinach, arugula, or baby kale)
- 1/3 cup Mexican vegan cheese, shredded
- 1/3 cup organic salsa
- 1 avocado, pitted and diced
- 1 handful of cilantro, washed and chopped
- ¼ cup plain coconut yogurt or dairy-free sour cream
- 1 lime, quartered

Instructions:

1. Combine all spices together in a small dish, stirring to combine. Set aside.

2. Prepare tomato, onion, cilantro and avocado and set aside

3. In a 10-inch cast-iron skillet, heat the oil for a few seconds. Add the ground beef to the skillet, cooking for 5-7 minutes until there's just a little bit of pink left. Remove from heat for a moment just to pour off excess liquid. Return to medium-low heat and stir taco seasoning in. Cook for another 2-3 minutes, stirring frequently until completely cooked. Remove from heat.

4. Layer the greens, followed by the taco meat and beans. Top with desired veggies and fix-ins.

*Eden Foods makes their beans with kombu by a pressure-cooking method. It removes anti-nutrients such as lectins that are usually found in beans and makes them easier to digest. You can also pressure-cook your own beans at home if you have an Instant Pot.

Mediterranean Chicken Salad with Honey Dijon Dressing

(Serves 2)

<u>Ingredients:</u>

- 6 cups mixed greens
- 1 red, orange and yellow bell peppers, chopped and lightly sautéed
- ½ cup edamame, shelled and cooked
- 1 large beet, cooked and sliced
- ¼ cup sheep's milk feta cheese, crumbled
- 1 cup chickpeas, cooked and drained (Eden Brand)
- ¼ red onion, finely diced
- 1 medium cucumber, chopped
- 1 pound free-range, organic chicken breast
- ½ teaspoon garlic powder
- Sea salt and pepper to taste
- 1 handful parsley, finely chopped

<u>Honey Dijon Dressing Ingredients:</u>

- 1/4 cup certified organic olive oil
- 1 tablespoon raw local honey
- 1 tablespoon Dijon mustard
- 1 clove garlic, minced
- 1/2 teaspoon dried oregano
- Salt and pepper to taste

<u>Instructions:</u>

1. Preheat the oven to 425 degrees F. Prepare a baking sheet with parchment paper. Season the chicken with garlic powder, salt and pepper. Bake for 15-18 minutes, flipping halfway through.

Remove from the oven when the internal temperature of the chicken reaches 160 degrees F.

2. While the chicken is baking, steam the beet by cutting it into 4 pieces and steaming it with ½ inch of water in a saucepan, covered. Steam for around 10 minutes until fork tender. Prepare the rest of the vegetables. When the chicken is done, let cool slightly and then chop into bite-sized pieces.

3. Combine ingredients for the dressing in a jar or measuring glass. Stir together until completely combined.

4. Assemble the salads by placing the greens on two large plates or bowls, followed by the rest of the vegetables and chicken. Drizzle the dressing over the surface of each salad and top with fresh parsley.

Seared Salmon with Mashed Cauliflower

(Serves 2)

Ingredients:

- 2 wild-caught, 1-inch thick Alaskan Salmon fillets
- ½ teaspoon garlic powder
- Sea salt and black pepper to taste
- 1 tablespoon certified organic olive oil
- 1 organic lemon

For the Cauliflower:

- 4 cups organic cauliflower, chopped into florets
- 1 tablespoon nutritional yeast
- ¼ teaspoon garlic powder
- ¼ teaspoon sea salt + more to taste
- 1/8 teaspoon black pepper + more to taste
- 2 tablespoons coconut yogurt
- Optional: 1 tablespoon freshly grated, raw parmesan cheese

Instructions:

1. Turn the oven to 425 degrees F. Turn a cast-iron skillet on medium-high heat, prepare salmon with salt, pepper, garlic powder. Coat the cast-iron skillet in olive oil, placing salmon in skillet skin-side up so the flesh meets the surface of the pan. Turn burner up to high and let sear for 2-3 min without turning. Then, take the whole skillet and place in the oven to bake for 6-10 min (Cook longer for thicker than 1-inch salmon fillets).

2. While the salmon is baking, place cauliflower florets in a medium saucepan with a lid and 1 inch of water. Turn on

medium-high and steam for around 10 minutes, or until the cauliflower is just fork-tender. Discard the any remaining water. Using tongs, place all the cauliflower florets into a high speed blender or food processor with the seasonings and yogurt. Pulse the blender, using a tamper to push the contents into the blades. If you don't have a tamper, periodically stop the blender or food processor and scrape the ingredients down the sides into the blades until completely smooth and incorporated. Taste and add more seasonings if desired.

3. Carefully remove cast-iron skillet with salmon from the oven with an oven mitt, take salmon out of the pan with a spatula and set aside.

4. Plate salmon and mashed cauliflower and squeeze fresh lemon juice over the tops of the salmon fillets.

Salmon Teriyaki Bowl (serves 2)

Adapted from Justin Schuble's Salmon Rice Bowl)

For the Marinated Salmon:

- 1 large Alaskan salmon filets, sliced into squares
- 1/4 cup coconut aminos
- 1/2 tsp garlic powder
- 2 tsp sriracha
- 2 tsp rice vinegar
- 1 spring onion thinly sliced
- 1/4 tsp ginger powder (or 2 teaspoons grated ginger)
- Toppings: sliced avocado, sesame seeds, seaweed flakes, fresh lime wedges

Cauliflower rice:

- 6 cups cauliflower rice
- 1 tbsp rice vinegar
- Sea salt

Sriracha mayo:

- 1 tbsp olive oil mayonnaise,
- 1 tsp rice vinegar
- 1 tsp sriracha

Instructions:

1. Turn oven on to 400 degrees F. Place salmon pieces in a flat dish with edges. Whisk marinade ingredients together in a bowl and pour over salmon, stir around and refrigerate for 30 minutes.

2. In a large pot, steam the cauliflower rice for 5-7 minutes with 1/4 cup water. Add the rice vinegar and a sprinkle of salt. Whisk together the sriracha mayonnaise and set aside.

3. Arrange the salmon pieces on a lined baking tray and bake for 8 min.

4. Layer the rice in a bowl followed by salmon, sliced avocado, sesame seeds, seaweed flakes, and fresh lime.

Roasted Red Pepper Soup

(Yields ~7 cups of soup, serves 3-4)

Ingredients:

- 1 tablespoon certified organic olive oil
- 3 red bell peppers, cored
- 4 roma tomatoes, quartered
- 1/2 cup basil leaves
- 5-6 small garlic cloves, peeled
- 1 medium sweet onion, quartered
- ¾ teaspoon sea salt + more to taste
- ¼ teaspoon freshly ground black pepper
- 1 handful fresh parsley
- 3/4 cup full fat, canned coconut milk
- 1 tablespoon nutritional yeast

Instructions:

1. Preheat the oven to 400 degrees F. Place bell peppers, tomatoes, garlic, and onion in a cast iron skillet. Bake in skillet for 30-35 minutes or until veggies are fork tender and are slightly browned.

2. Place veggies, nutritional yeast, parsley, basil, coconut milk, salt, and pepper in a high-speed blender. Blend for 30 seconds, using a tamper to push the contents into the blades. Taste soup and add extra basil or sea salt and pepper if you prefer.

3. Pour into a bowl or mug and top with sliced basil and a dollop of coconut cream. Enjoy immediately with a slice of your favorite sourdough bread.

∼

STEAK AND VEGGIE FAJITA BOWL

(Serves 2)

Ingredients:

- 2 tablespoons certified organic olive oil
- 1 medium green bell pepper, thinly sliced
- 1 medium yellow bell pepper, thinly sliced
- 1 medium red bell pepper, thinly sliced
- ½ white onion, thinly sliced
- 10 ounces grass-fed steak
- ½ teaspoon garlic powder
- Sea salt and pepper
- 1 handful fresh cilantro, chopped
- Serving suggestions: Serve with brown rice and black beans and top with chopped cilantro, dairy-free cheese, sour cream, and salsa, and avocado

Instructions:

1. Preheat a large cast-iron skillet on medium heat. Add 1 tablespoon of olive oil and let heat slightly before adding the onion to the pan. Let onion cook for 3 minutes, then add the bell peppers and saute for 3-5 minutes, until just fork tender. Remove from the skillet and set aside.

2. While veggies are sautéing, season both sides of the steak with garlic powder, salt and pepper. Preheat a separate cast-iron skillet to medium-high heat, and add the rest of the olive oil and let heat slightly. Add the steak to the pan and cook for 4-5 minutes on each side, cooking to preferred tenderness level.

3. Once the steak is cooked, slice with a steak knife into thin strips. Distribute the sides, veggies and steak evenly between two plates and add toppings.

MUSHROOM PROTEIN BOWL

(Serves 2)

Ingredients:

- 1 tablespoon certified organic olive oil
- 2 cloves of garlic, minced
- 10 ounces cremini mushrooms
- 6 ounces organic ground turkey
- 3/4 teaspoon sea salt
- Freshly ground black pepper to taste
- 1/2 teaspoon dried basil
- 6 ounces kale, torn into pieces
- 1 can organic chickpeas (Eden brand)
- 1/3 cup full fat, canned coconut milk
- 1 1/2 tablespoons nutritional yeast
- Optional: 1 teaspoon freshly squeezed lemon juice, freshly grated raw parmesan cheese for topping

Instructions:

1. Heat a large cast-iron skill to medium low heat, add the olive oil and garlic. Sauté until slightly browned and fragrant.

2. Add in the mushrooms and cook for 4 minutes, followed by ground turkey, salt, pepper, and basil. Cook until there is just a small amount of pink remaining. Add the kale and stir. Pour in coconut milk and nutritional yeast, and lemon juice. stir to incorporate. Bring to a simmer for 3-4 min. Remove from heat.

3. Using a ladle, spoon into 2 separate bowls, add the chickpeas, and top with freshly grated parmesan cheese.

Curry Chicken Salad

(Makes 3-4 servings)

Ingredients:

- 1-pound free-range, organic chicken breast
- 1/2 cup olive oil or avocado oil mayonnaise
- 2 tablespoons coconut yogurt
- 1/2 green apple, diced
- 1/4 red onion diced
- 2 tablespoons unsweetened dried cranberries, chopped
- 1/2 teaspoons sea salt + more for seasoning the chicken
- ½ and ¼ teaspoons garlic powder
- 1 tablespoon curry powder
- 1/8 teaspoon onion powder
- 2 teaspoons Dijon mustard
- Freshly ground black pepper, to taste

Instructions:

1. Preheat the oven to 425 degrees F. Prepare a baking sheet with parchment paper. Season the chicken with ½ teaspoon garlic powder, and salt and pepper to taste. Bake for 15-18 minutes, flipping halfway through. Remove from the oven when the internal temperature of the chicken reaches 160 degrees F.

2. While the chicken is baking, slice the apple and cranberries. Add these, the yogurt, mayonnaise, remaining spices, and mustard to a large mixing bowl.

3. When the chicken has cooled slightly, chop into smaller than bite-sized pieces and add to the mixing bowl. Stir to combine.

4. Enjoy as a sandwich on sourdough bread, lettuce-wrapped, or as a salad topper on a bed of baby kale mixed greens.

Turkey Burgers with Sweet Potato Fries

(Makes 4 burgers)

For the burgers:

- 1 tablespoon organic olive oil
- 1-pound organic ground turkey
- 1 large free-range, organic egg
- 2 cloves garlic, minced or grated
- ¼ cup sweet yellow onion, finely chopped
- 1 teaspoon dried basil
- ½ teaspoon dried oregano
- ¼ teaspoon black pepper
- ¾ teaspoon sea salt

For the fries:

(Recipe by Mark Bittman)

- 1-pound organic sweet potatoes
- 1 tablespoon organic olive oil
- ½ teaspoon sea salt
- ½ teaspoon black pepper
- ½ teaspoon paprika
- ½ teaspoon garlic powder

Special Dipping Sauce:

- ¼ cup avocado oil mayonnaise
- 1 teaspoon yellow mustard
- 1 tablespoon organic, sugar-free ketchup
- ¼ teaspoon garlic powder
- A pinch of sea salt

Side suggestions: Romaine lettuce leaves, tomato, ketchup, mustard, pickles, sliced onion.

Instructions:

1. Preheat the oven to 400 degrees F. Prepare a large baking sheet with parchment paper and set aside. Slice the sweet potatoes into wedges that are about ¼ inch thick. In a large mixing bowl, combine the olive oil and sweet potatoes. Toss the sweet potatoes with a spatula to coat them in oil. Pour the seasonings into the bowl and mix to coat each sweet potato wedge. Lay the wedges on the baking sheet in a single layer. Bake for 15 minutes, flipping and then baking for another 10 minutes.

2. While the sweet potatoes fries are baking, combine all ingredients for the burgers in a large mixing bowl. Mix until a uniform mixture forms. Separate into 4 sections and form into patties. Heat the olive oil in a large cast-iron skillet and cook each burger for 4-5 minutes on each side, flipping only once. Cook until the burgers reach an internal temperature of 160 degrees F.

3. Combine all ingredients for the special dipping sauce in a jar or a bowl and set aside. Arrange the fries, burger patties, and vegetable sides on plates and serve.

GRASS-FED GROUND BEEF, VEGGIE, AND QUINOA BOWL

(Serves 2-3)

Ingredients:

- 1 tablespoon organic olive oil
- ¼ white onion, sliced
- 1 clove garlic, peeled and minced
- 2 cups chopped asparagus stalks
- 2 cups butternut squash, diced
- 1-pound grass-fed ground beef
- 1 teaspoon sea salt
- ¼ teaspoon black pepper
- ½ teaspoon dried basil
- 1 cup organic dry sprouted quinoa
- Dairy-free ranch dressing*

Instructions:

1. Prepare quinoa according to the package instructions.

2. Heat olive oil in a large, cast-iron skillet. Add the garlic and saute for 30 seconds or until slightly browned and fragrant. Add the onion to the skillet and saute for about 3 minutes, or until slightly translucent. Add the butternut squash and asparagus to the skillet and cover for about 2 minutes.

3. Add the ground beef and spices and mix thoroughly to combine everything. Stir every few minutes, covering in between. Cook until the pink has completely disappeared from the beef. Serve with quinoa and top with dairy-free ranch.

*Recipe found in the bonus PDF or purchase Primal Kitchen ranch dressing

CRISPY ALMOND FLOUR CRUST PIZZA

(Serves 2-3)

Crust:

- 2 cups blanched almond flour
- ½ teaspoon sea salt
- 1 teaspoon baking soda
- 1 teaspoon garlic powder
- 1 organic large egg

Toppings:

- ½ cup low-sugar marinara sauce
- 1 ½ cups vegan mozzarella shredded cheese**
- ½ teaspoon dried basil
- ½ teaspoon dried oregano

Additional toppings: Turkey pepperoni, bell peppers, black olives, chicken, anchovies, basil

Instructions:

1. Preheat the oven to 400 degrees F. Line a large baking sheet or pizza baking sheet with parchment paper. In a large bowl, whisk almond flour, salt, baking soda, and garlic powder together. Whisk the egg in a separate small bowl. Mix the egg into the almond flour mixture with a spatula until a smooth, uniform dough forms. If the dough is too crumbly, add a tablespoon of water to it.

2. Transfer the dough to the baking sheet and cover it with another sheet of parchment paper. Using a rolling pin, flatten

the dough by rolling it into a large circle that is about ¼ inch thick. Take the top parchment paper off.

3. Bake the crust in the oven for about 7-8 minutes, and the edges are just beginning to brown. Remove from the oven.

4. Spoon the sauce onto the partially baked crust and spreading it thin. Sprinkle the cheese evenly around, followed by the spices and desired toppings.

5. Bake the pizza in the oven again until the cheese has melted (5-10 minutes). Remove and allow to cool slightly, then slicing as desired with a pizza cutter.

*May substitute for 1 ¼ cup shredded raw mozzarella cheese + ¼ cup shredded raw parmesan cheese (Pizza crust recipe by Vered DeLeeuw)

Cheesy Butternut Squash Bowl with Cooked Quinoa

(Makes 2-3 servings)

Ingredients:

- 4 cups butternut squash, sliced into ¼ inch by 2-inch sticks
- 1 cup zucchini, sliced
- 1 cup baby Bella mushrooms, sliced
- 1 yellow onion, sliced
- 2 cloves garlic, minced
- 1 tablespoon avocado oil
- 1 pound organic, pasture-raised chicken breast
- ½ teaspoon garlic powder
- Sea salt and pepper to taste
- 1/4 cup nutritional yeast
- Optional: ¼ teaspoon turmeric powder for color
- 1 cup unsweetened nut milk from a carton*
- 1/4 cup canned coconut milk
- 1 cup sprouted quinoa, measured dry
- Optional: Freshly grated, raw Parmesan cheese

Instructions:

1. Turn oven on to 425 degrees F and prepare a baking sheet with parchment paper. Rinse quinoa before placing in the instant pot with water. Sprinkle a little sea salt in if desired. Cook quinoa in an Instant Pot on manual, high pressure for 3 minutes, allowing a natural release for 11 minutes at the end of the cooking cycle.

2. Season chicken breast with garlic powder, salt and pepper on both sides, then bake for 15-18 minutes, flipping halfway through. Remove from oven and let cool.

3. In a large cast-iron skillet, heat olive oil slightly, then add the garlic and sauce for 30 seconds. Add the followed by mushrooms and onions. Let sauté for 4-5 minutes, then add the butternut squash. Cover and cook for 3 minutes. Then, add zucchini, cooking another 3 minutes. Remove from heat when all veggies are fork-tender.

4. Combine approximately 1/2 the cooked onion and around 1 cup of the cooked butternut squash from the skillet inside a large high-speed blender pitcher. Pour in nutritional yeast, salt/pepper to taste, and milk in the blender. Blend on high for 30 seconds until smooth. Taste and add more seasonings to your preference.

5. Cut chicken breast into bite-sized chunks, and plate with the veggies and quinoa in separate bowls. Pour sauce over the top, sprinkle with fresh parmesan cheese if desired and enjoy!

~

<u>Snack and Dessert Recipes</u>

GRAIN-FREE CHOCOLATE CHIP COOKIES (GLUTEN-FREE, DAIRY-FREE, SUGAR-FREE)

(Yields approximately 24 cookies)

<u>Ingredients:</u>

- 2 large eggs
- 1/2 cup allulose
- 1/2 teaspoon Red Sea salt
- 1/2 teaspoon baking soda
- 1 teaspoon vanilla extract
- 1/3 cup coconut oil
- 3 cups blanched almond flour
- 1/2 cup sugar-free, dairy-free chocolate chips

<u>Instructions:</u>

1. Preheat oven to 375 degrees F and prep 2 baking pans with parchment paper and set aside.

2. In a medium mixing bowl, combine eggs, sweetener, salt, baking soda and vanilla extract. Mix with an electric mixer until combined. Add coconut oil and mix again until incorporated. Add almond flour 1 cup at a time, using a spatula when it gets too thick for the mixer. Add in most of the chocolate chips, saving a few for topping.

3. Scoop cookie dough with a scoop or 2 spoons. You can also roll with your hands. Place on cookie sheet 2 inches apart, top with remaining chocolate chips. Bake for 10-15 min until edges

are golden brown. Let cool on baking tray for 10 min, then transfer to cooling rack.

~

HEALTHY CHOCOLATE ZUCCHINI BREAD (GLUTEN-FREE, DAIRY-FREE, SUGAR-FREE)

(Yields 8-10 slices)

Ingredients:

- 2 organic, pasture-raised eggs
- 2/3 cup allulose
- 1/2 cup cacao powder
- 1 tablespoon melted extra-virgin, organic coconut oil
- 1 cup almond flour
- 1 serving of chocolate protein powder or collagen
- ¼ cup unsweetened hemp seed milk
- 2/3 cup shredded zucchini
- 1/4 cup sugar-free, dairy-free dark chocolate chips

Instructions:

1. Preheat your oven to 375 degrees F and line a 9x5 inch loaf pan with parchment paper. In large mixing bowl, stir all ingredients together except for the shredded zucchini and chocolate chips. Once completely combined and smooth, add them in.

2. Pour into the baking dish and bake for 25-30 minutes. Remove from the oven when a toothpick comes out clean.

3. Let cool slightly for 20 minutes, then remove from the pan and let cool completely on a baking rack. Slice and serve.

Healthy Chocolate Pudding (gluten-free, sugar-free, dairy-free)

(Makes two 3 oz servings)

Ingredients:

- 1/2 cup unsweetened nut or seed milk
- 1 tablespoon granulated monk fruit sweetener
- 1 ½ oz sugar-free 85% dark chocolate baking bar or chocolate chips
- 1/4 cup cacao powder
- 1 teaspoon agar-agar powder*
- Optional add-in: ½ serving chocolate bone broth protein**
- Optional toppings: Freeze-dried strawberries or chopped raspberries, sea salt

Instructions:

1. Place pieces of chocolate in a medium glass measuring cup or mixing bowl. Bring the milk and sweetener to a boil, stirring frequently.

2. Remove from heat once it comes to a boil. Pour the mixture over the chocolate and let sit 30 seconds before stirring. Whisk until combined, then add in the cacao powder, protein powder (if using) and sprinkle agar-agar over the surface, whisking until all clumps dissolve. The mixture should be liquid-consistency or slightly thicker than.

3. Let the mixture cool at room temperature for 30 minutes, and then transfer to the fridge for 4 hours to set. Top with fruit and sea salt before enjoying.

*Agar-agar is a plant-based gelatin that comes from seaweed.

**Adds in an extra protein source and makes the pudding more filling. If using protein powder, use 3 tablespoons cacao powder instead of ¼ cup.

~

ALMOND BUTTER CUPS

(Makes 6 cups)

Ingredients:

- 1/2 cup natural almond butter
- 1 teaspoon vanilla extract
- 1/2 teaspoon almond extract
- 3 tablespoons monk fruit maple syrup
- 1/4 cup vanilla protein powder or collagen powder
- 1 tablespoon coconut flour
- ¾ cup dairy-free chocolate chips
- 2 teaspoons coconut oil
- Coarse sea salt for topping

Instructions:

1. Line a 6-muffin tin with paper muffin liners or use a silicone mold. Combine almond butter, extracts, syrup, protein powder, and coconut flour in a medium mixing bowl until incorporated. Distribute batter evenly across all cups. Press firmly into the bases. Set aside.

2. Melt the chocolate and coconut oil over a water bath or in the microwave until smooth, stirring frequently. Pour over the tops of the cups, distributing evenly. Sprinkle with coarse sea salt. Let set in the fridge for at least 30 min to solidify.

BLUEBERRY CARDAMOM MUFFINS

(Makes ~12-16 muffins)

Ingredients:

- 2 eggs, beaten
- 1 cup plain coconut yogurt or Greek yogurt
- 1/2 cup coconut oil, melted
- 1/2 tsp vanilla extract
- 1/3 cup coconut flour
- 1 cup almond flour
- 1 ½ cups allulose
- 1/2 tsp baking powder
- 1/2 tsp baking soda
- 1/2 tsp sea salt
- 1 teaspoon dried cardamom
- 1 1/2 cups fresh blueberries

Instructions:

1. Preheat the oven to 350 degrees F. Prepare a 12-muffin pan with coconut oil or avocado oil cooking spray and muffin liners.

2. Using an electric whisk, mix all wet ingredients together in a large mixing bowl. Add the dry ingredients and whisk to combine. Fold in the blueberries.

3. Spoon the batter into muffin sections. Bake for 15-22 minutes, until the tops are golden brown and a toothpick comes out clean. Let cool for about 20 minutes in the mold and then transfer to a baking rack. Enjoy while warm.

Healthy Banana Pudding (with Homemade Vanilla Wafers)

(Makes 2 servings)

Banana Pudding Ingredients:

- 1 large, ripe banana, mashed
- 2 tablespoons probiotic cream cheese, softened*
- 1/4 cup plain Greek yogurt**
- ½ serving vanilla protein powder
- 1/2 teaspoon vanilla extract
- 1/4 teaspoon almond extract
- 2 tablespoons powdered monk fruit extract
- 1/3 cup of coconut whipped cream (need 1 can of full-fat coconut milk, see below)

Vanilla Wafer Ingredients:

- ½ cup gluten-free flour*
- 1/2 cup almond flour
- 1/3 cup powdered monk fruit sweetener
- ¾ teaspoon baking powder
- pinch of sea salt
- 2 tablespoons coconut oil
- 1 tablespoon vanilla extract
- 1 medium egg
- 1 tablespoon unsweetened nut milk

Instructions:

1. Put a can of coconut milk in the fridge overnight to allow the cream to separate. Don't shake the can or mix it.

2. For the wafers, preheat the oven to 350 degrees F. Line a baking sheet with parchment paper.

3. Mix dry ingredients for the wafers in a large mixing bowl, followed by the wet ingredients. Combine until a dough forms.

4. Form the dough into small balls in the size of about ~ 1/2 tablespoon in your hands. Place them on the baking sheet, and flatten them with the back of a spoon or spatula. Bake for 12-15 min, until slightly golden-brown edges. Let cool on the pan slightly and then set aside on a rack.

5. While the wafers are baking, remove the lid from the coconut milk, being careful not to shake it. Scoop the top layer of cream out of the can with a spoon and place in a large, chilled mixing bowl. Whip the coconut milk solids with an electric mixer until light and fluffy. Set aside.

6. For the banana pudding, mash the banana, then add all ingredients together except whipped cream. Whisk with an electric mixer until incorporated, then fold in the whipped cream at the end with a spatula.

7. Crush some wafers and layer them in the bottom of a glass and banana slices if desired. Layer in banana pudding, followed by more whipped cream, crumbled wafers and banana slices. Repeat until the glass is full. Topping suggestions: Additional coconut whipped cream and sliced banana.

*Purchase your own in the store, or make this <u>DIY Gluten-Free Flour Blend:</u>

- 1 tablespoon tapioca flour
- 1 tbsp coconut flour
- 6 tablespoons oat flour

DOWNLOAD THE BONUS PDF TO THIS BOOK FOR FULL SUPPORT

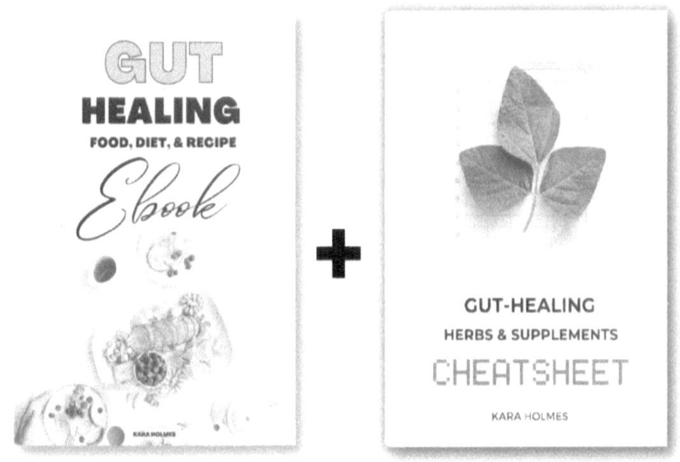

Scan the QR code to get:

- **Worksheets** to help you implement new habits and track your progress.

- **The Beginner's Guide to Gut-Healing Herbs and Supplements,** which will answer all your remaining questions about supplementing for gut health.
- **Over twenty additional gut-friendly recipes,** including comfort food, coffee, and desserts.
- A comprehensive, **gut-healthy grocery list.**
- A **color PDF** of the Gut Healing Plan that you can print out.
- A list of **clever, gut-healthy food and snack swaps.**

https://vitalitycoaching.org/guthealthresetbonuses/

A QUICK REVIEW HELPS OTHERS

Hi there! I just wanted to check in and ask how you enjoyed the book? I would be incredibly thankful if you took sixty seconds to leave a quick review on Amazon, even if it's just a sentence or two. Many readers don't know how hard reviews are to come by, and how much they help other people looking for the right book when starting their gut-healing journey. Scan the QR code below with your phone camera, or simply head to the Orders section while logged into your Amazon profile and you'll see this book. Click on the book and then it will show you an option to leave a review. It's that simple! I look forward to reading your review. You can leave me a little message as well, as I personally read and appreciate every review.

RESOURCES

Scan the QR code to access links when reading paperback and hardcover versions of this book:

Note: There are some affiliate links included in the bonus PDF and the supplement recommendations. I only recommend products I've tried myself and that I know are effective. Your support is always appreciated.

Providers & 1:1 Support

Book a Free 1:1 Gut Health and Nutrition Coaching Session with Kara Holmes. Coaching and nutrition counseling are available over video or phone call.– https://vitalitycoaching.org/contact/

Find a Functional Medicine Provider: https://www.ifm.org/find-a-practitioner/

Ideal Bodies Nutrition (Offers virtual and in-person consultations in the Los Angeles area: https://www.idealbodiesnutrition.com/

Recommended Probiotics:

Plexus Probio5 – Great for candida overgrowth and balancing out helpful gut flora. It's lower potency and is a good starter probiotic.

Plexus VitalBiome – A step up from Probio5 and with strains that have been clinically researched regarding how they support mental health.

Seed DS-01™ Daily Synbiotic – One of the most comprehensive and valuable probiotics on the market. The strains inside have been tested for effective mental health improvement, weight management, skin, and hormone health.

Other Recommendations:

Triplex for Gut Restoration – A high quality system to eradicate SIBO/SIFO, yeast, and candida overgrowth. Helps rebalance gut flora while supporting stable appetite and blood sugar balance. This helped me recover from prediabetes, disordered eating, candida, and leaky gut, as well as lose thirty pounds. I used it for five months in total, then weaned off it.

CandiBactin AR and Candibactin BR - A well-researched, highly approved supplement to eradicate SIBO and SIFO. Together, these herbal formulations work to reduce harmful bacteria, fungi, and candida so helpful bacteria can repopulate.

Note: When supplementing for SIBO, it's helpful to consult with a provider. For a full list of recommended supplements, doses, and where to find them affordably, check the bonus PDF guide, a gift to you for purchasing this book.

Lab Testing:

Request a Test – Have you ever been curious about your mineral, cholesterol, blood sugar, or triglyceride levels? These results can be obtained by running a sample of your blood. Now, you don't need a doctor to order the test for you. Simply order tests yourself and get the result, with the option to forward it to your doctor. https://requestatest.com/

Breath Test for All SIBO Types:

This breath testing meter tests for the presence of all gases that can exist with SIBO, making it the most comprehensive.

www.triosmartbreath.com/orderonline

Check Out My Other Books on Amazon:

- Freed and Fierce: the 7 Untapped Essentials for Life-Long Eating Disorder Recovery

- The Anxiety Relief Coloring Book for Adults

Scan the QR code to access these books

NOTES

1. Why Is the Gut Important?

1. See Sunrise Hospital & Medical Center (2017) for more information on gut health and preventing disease.
2. See Harvard Health (2016) for more information on gut bacteria improving your health.
3. Shreiner, A. B., Kao, J. Y., & Young, V. B. (2015). The gut microbiome in health and in disease.
4. See Ellis, J. L., Karl, J. P. (2021) for more information on vitamins and the gut microbiome.
5. See Morowitz, M. J., Carlisle, E. M. (2011) for more information on gut bacteria and B-12 synthesis.
6. See Petersen, C., & Round, J. L. (2014) for more information on defining gut dysbiosis.
7. See Petersen, C., & Round, J. L. (2014) for more information on defining gut dysbiosis
8. See Frederick Health (2021) for more information on symptoms of poor gut health
9. See Frederick Health (2021) for more information on symptoms of poor gut health

2. Looking at the Inside: Digestive System 101

1. See Stool Changes and What They Mean. (2019) for more information on digestive patterns
2. See Stool Changes and What They Mean. (2019) for more information on digestive patterns.

3. Do You Have a Higher Risk of Gut Dysbiosis?

1. See Neu, J., & Rushing, J. (2011) for more information about cesarean versus vaginal delivery.
2. See Shao, Y., (2019) for more information about the cesarean delivery microbiome research study.

3. See the Centers for Disease Control (2021) for more information on hospital-acquired infections.

4. See Żukiewicz-Sobczak, W., (2014) for more information on lactic acid bacteria and prevention of allergy and disease.

5. See Naleway A. L. (2004) for more information on asthma, farming, and the immune system.

6. See Klintberg, B., Berglund, N (2001) for more information on asthma, the immune system and farming.

7. See Satokari R. (2020) for more information about refined foods and the gut microbiome

8. See Bian, X., Tu, P., (2017) for more information on saccharin and blood sugar, and gut health.

9. See Tu, P., Chi, L., (2020) for more information about gut health and artificial sweeteners.

10. See Meroni, M., Longo, M., & Dongiovanni, P. (2019) for more information on alcohol and the gut microbiome.

11. See Amen, D.G, (2013 for more information on antibiotics and food

12. See Khalili H. (2016) for more information on oral contraceptives and gut health

13. See Khalili H. (2016) for more information on oral contraceptives and gut health

14. *See Hypochlorhydria (Low Stomach Acid* - Cleveland Clinic 2022) for more information on low stomach acid.

15. See Breton, J. (2013) for more information on heavy metals and the gut microbiome.

16. See Heavy Metals | The Caribbean environment programme (2008) for more information on heavy metals.

17. See Rafati Rahimzadeh, M.(2017) for more information on cadmium toxicity.

18. See Balali-Mood, M. (2021) for more information on heavy metal toxicity.

19. See Heavy Metals | The Caribbean environment programme (2008) for more information on heavy metals.

20. See Balali-Mood, M. (2021) for more information on heavy metal toxicity.

21. See Liu, T., Liang, X., (2020) for more information on the gut microbiome and heavy metal detoxification.

22. See Harris, L. (2021) for more information on gut health and microplastics.

23. See Huang, Z., & Weng,Y. (2021) for more information on microplastics and the gut

24. See *11 Safest Non Toxic Cookware Brands For A Healthy Kitchen in 2022.* (n.d.). for more information

25. See *11 Safest Non Toxic Cookware Brands For A Healthy Kitchen in 2022.* (n.d.). for more information

26. See Tu, P., Chi, L., (2020) for more information about gut health and pesticides

27. See Glenny, E.M. (2017) for more information on gut health and eating disorders.

28. See van Hoeken, D., & Hoek, H. W. (2020) for more information on morbidity of eating disorders.

4. Understanding IBS, SIBO / SIFO, and Leaky Gut Syndrome

1. See Weaver, K. R., Melkus, G. D., & Henderson, W. A. (2017) for more information on IBS.

2. See Appleton J. (2018) for more information on the gut-brain axis, GI and mental health.

3. See Achufusi, T., Sharma, A., Zamora, E. A., & Manocha, D. (2020) for more information in SIBO.

4. See *Small intestinal bacterial overgrowth (SIBO) - Symptoms and causes* (2022) for more information.

5. See *Small intestinal bacterial overgrowth (SIBO) - Symptoms and causes* (2022) for more information.

6. See Rao, S., Tan, G. (2018) for more information on SIBO and colectomy surgery.

7. See Kim, D. B., Paik, C. N. (2018) for more information on gallbladder disease and SIBO.

8. See Roberts, M. (2020) for more information on supporting bile flow.

9. See Gaci, N., Borrel, G. (2014) for more information on SIBO, Archaea and breath testing.

10. See *Colonoscopy - Everything you need to know about the procedure.* (n.d.). Retrieved September 9, 2022 for more information on colonoscopes.

11. See *Endoscopy.* (2022, August 22). Merck Manuals for more information on endoscopes.

12. See *Testing.* (n.d.). SIBO - Small Intestine Bacterial Overgrowth. Retrieved September 9, 2022 for more information on endoscopy and testing for SIBO.

13. See Rao, S., & Bhagatwala, J. (2019) for more information on antibiotics and SIBO treatment.

14. See *Rifaximin (Oral Route).* (2022, February 14) Retrieved September 9, 2022 for more information.

15. See GoodRx.com "Rifaximin" (Retrieved Sept, 2022) https://www.goodrx.-com/rifaximin for more information.

16. See Saadi, M., & McCallum, R. W. (2013). For more information on Rifaximin and re-treatment rates.

17. See Chedid, V., Dhalla, S. (2014) for more information on SIBO and herbal remedies.

18. See Zardast, M., Namakin, K., (2016) for more information on garlic and H. pylori.

19. See Ansary, J., Forbes-Hernández, T. Y. (2020) for more information on garlic uses in conditions.

20. See Lopresti, A. L., Smith, S. J., Rea, A., & Michel, S. (2021) for more information on curcumin IBS, and SIBO.

21. See Miller, A. L., Bessho, S., Grando, K., & Tükel, Ç. (2021) for more information on bacterial colonies and biofilms.

22. See Lane, A., Dalkie, N., Henderson, L., Irwin, J., & Rostami, K. (2021) for more information on the Elemental diet.

23. See Patterson, R. E., Laughlin, G. A. (2015) for more information on intermittent fasting and chronic disease.

24. See Patterson, R. E., Laughlin, G. A. (2015) for more information on intermittent fasting and chronic disease.

25. See Collier R. (2013) for more information on (IF) and cellular resilience.

26. See Mohr, A. E., (2021) for more information on intermittent fasting.

27. See Toro-Londono, M. A. (2019) for more information on parasitic infections.

28. See Head K. A. (2008) for more information on berberine and parasitic infections.

29. See Meroni, M. (2019) for more information on helpful gut bacteria populations and the impact on leaky gut.

30. See Caricilli, A. M., Castoldi, A., (2014) for more information on the intestinal barrier and the immune system.

31. See Caricilli, A. M., Castoldi, A., (2014) for more information on the intestinal barrier and the immune system.

32. See Furman, D., Campisi, J. (2019 for more information on the relationship between inflammation, disease, and the intestinal barrier.

33. See Sunrise Hospital & Medical Center (2017) for more information on promoting optimal gut health and preventing disease.

34. See Shankle, W. R., & M.D., D. A. G. (2005) for more information on preventing Alzheimer's disease.

35. See the Society for Endocrinology (2017) for more information on corticotrophin-releasing hormone.

36. See the Society for Endocrinology (2017) for more information on corticotrophin-releasing hormone.

37. See Bertani, B., & Ruiz, N. (2018) for more information on LPS and cellular permeability.

38. See Ngkelo, A. (2012, January 12) for more information on LPS.

39. See Hollon, J., (2015) for more information on zonulin, gliadin and intestinal permeability.

40. See Fasano A. (2012) for more information on zonulin and intestinal permeability.
41. See Drago, S., El Asmar, R. (2006) for more information on zonulin, gliadin, and intestinal permeability.
42. See the Simplified Guide to the Gut-Brain Axis (October 2021) for more information about how the gut talks to the brain.
43. See Bundgaard-Nielsen, C. (2020) for more information on the autism, ADD and the gut microbiome.
44. See Amen, D.G. (2013) for more information on ADD and autism and the gut microbiome.
45. See Ma, T., Jin, H., Kwok, L. Y., Sun, Z., Liong, M. T., & Zhang, H. (2021) for more information on probiotics and improvement in depression and anxiety.
46. See Lew, L. (2019) for more information on probiotics and improvement in depression and anxiety.

5. Lifestyle Foundations for Supporting a Healthy Gut

1. See Akimbekov, N. S. (2020) for more information on Vitamin D and gut health.
2. See Thaiss, C. A., Zeevi, D. (2014) for more information on disruption in circadian rhythm and gut health.
3. See Takahashi T. (2012) for more information on the migrating motor complex.
4. See Lee, D. Y. (2022) for more information on IBD and vitamin and mineral deficiencies
5. See DiNicolantonio, J. J., O'Keefe, J. H., & Wilson, W. (2018) for more information on magnesium deficiency.
6. See Hijikata, Y., & Yamada, S. (2011) for more information on walking after dinner.
7. Monda, V., Villano, I. (2017) for more information on exercise and gut microbiota.
8. See Monda, V., Villano, I. (2017) for more information on exercise and gut microbiota.
9. See Reynolds, A. N., & Venn, B. J. (2018) for more information on blood sugar and physical activity.
10. See Madison, A., & Kiecolt-Glaser, J. K. (2019) for more information on stress and the gut microbiota.
11. See Househam, A. M., Peterson, C. T., Mills, P. J., & Chopra, D. (2017) for more information on stress management techniques for gut health.
12. See Madison, A., & Kiecolt-Glaser, J. K. (2019) for more information on stress, the gut, and exercise.

13. See Harvard Health. (2016a, June 16). Loneliness for more information on loneliness as a risk factor for heart disease.

6. Food Misconceptions: Have We Been Misled About Healthy Eating All Along?

1. See Sender, R., Fuchs, S., (2016) for more information on ratio of bacterial cells to human cells in the body.
2. See Rinninella, E. (2019) for more information on gut health, food, and chronic disease.
3. See Nestle, M. (2018) for more information about food marketing and health claims.
4. See Center for Food Safety and Applied Nutrition (2017, December 7) for more information on regulation of health claims in marketing.
5. See Ordovas, J.M. (2018) for more information on personalized nutrition and optimized wellness.
6. See *Obesity and overweight* (2021, June 9) The World Health Organization for more information on worldwide obesity and undernutrition.
7. See La Berge, A. F. (2007) for more information on the history of low-fat diets and public health
8. See La Berge, A. F. (2007) for more information on the history the American Heart Association and heart-healthy food labeling
9. See *Obesity and overweight* (2021) The World Health Organization for more information on obesity and malnutrition
10. See Rygiel K. (2018) for more information on HDL, LDL, and atherosclerosis.

7. Understanding How to Eat for a Healthy Gut

1. See Wang, P.X. (2020) for more information on gut health and metabolic syndrome.
2. See Lotta, L. A., Abbasi, A., (2015) for more information on metabolic health and heart disease.
3. See Ginsberg H. N. (2000). Insulin resistance and cardiovascular disease.
4. See Washington State University (n.d.). *Nutrition Basics* for more information on macronutrients.
5. See Rinninella, E., Cintoni, M. (2019) for more information on fiber and gut bacteria
6. See The Neurobiology of Substance Use, Misuse, and Addiction (2016) for more information on sugar and the brain.
7. See Martins, N., Ferreira, I. C. (2014) for more information on candida and sugar.

8. See Rinninella, E., Cintoni, M. (2019) for more information on sugar and gut bacteria.

9. See *Carbohydrates and Blood Sugar* (2016) for more information on glycemic index and carbohydrates.

10. See Glycemic Index of the Foods (2020) *GI of Cocoa Pops puffed Rice* for more information on glycemic index of cereal.

11. See Carbohydrates and Blood Sugar by Harvard (2016) for more information on glycemic index of food.

12. See Yang, Z., & Liao, S. F. (2019) for more information on amino acids and gut health.

13. See Biwas (2014) for more information on glutamine food sources.

14. See Carbone, J. W., & Pasiakos, S. M. (2019) for more information on protein and organ health.

15. See Diether, N., & Willing, B. (2019) for more information on how a diet high in protein influences the gut.

16. See Abrahams, M., O'Grady, R., & Prawitt, J. (2022) for more information on collagen and gut health.

17. See Nutrition, G. B. (2020) for more information on Omega-3's and gut health.

18. See Dyerberg, J., Madsen, P., (2010) for more information on omega-3 supplements.

19. See Jariwalla R.J., and Lalezari J. (2008) for more information on ALA and glutathione.

20. See the Office of Dietary Supplements - Omega-3 Fatty Acids (2022) for more information on omega-3 fatty acids.

21. See DiNicolantonio, J. J., & O'Keefe, J. H. (2017) for more information on PUFAS and obesity risk.

22. See Simopoulos, A. (2016)) for more information on recommended ratio of omega-3 to omega-6 fatty acids.

23. See Simopoulos, A. (2006) for more information on recommended omega-3 and omega-6 fatty acid ratio.

24. See Daley, C. A., Abbott, A. (2010) for more information on grass-fed versus grain-fed animals and saturated fat quality

25. See Astrup, A., Teicholz, N (2021) for more information on saturated fat and cardiovascular disease.

26. See Uhde, M., Ajamian, M., (2016) for more information on gluten and inflammation in the gut.

27. See Mullins, A. P., & Arjmandi, B. H. (2021) for more information on the health benefits of legumes.

28. See Panacer, K., & Whorwell, P. J. (2019) for more information on lectins.

29. See Aslam, H., Marx, W. (2020) for more information on dairy and gut health.

30. See Martins, N., Ferreira, I. C., (2014) for more information on refined sugar and candida.

31. See Fajstova, A., Galanova, N. (2020) for more information on sugar and health.
32. See Bellini, M., Tonarelli, S., (2020) for more information on FODMAPS and digestive health.

8. Food Allergies, Intolerances, and Sensitivities

1. See Żukiewicz-Sobczak, W., (2014) for more information on lactic acid bacteria and prevention of allergy and disease.
2. See Furman, D., Campisi, J. (2019) for more information on inflammation.
3. See Histamine Tolerance Awareness (2020) for more information about high histamine foods and gut health.
4. See the difference between celiac disease and gluten intolerance (2018) for more information.
5. See *Unproven Diagnostic Tests*. (n.d.). FoodAllergy.org. Retrieved September 7, 2022 for more information on unproven diagnostic tests for food allergies.
6. See Food Allergy Diagnosis and Testing, n.d. for more information on diagnosing food allergies.
7. See Cuthbert & Goodheart, 2007 for more information on muscle-testing and food sensitivities.
8. See The Gut Healing Ninja (2021). For more information on healing food sensitivities.

9. Probiotics and Supplements for Gut Health

1. See Sanders, M. E. (2011) for more information on the benefits of probiotics.
2. See Derrien, M., & van Hylckama Vlieg, J. E. (June) for more information on host benefits from probiotics.
3. See Fenster, K., Freeburg, B. (2019) for more information on probiotic viability.
4. See Gaon, D., Garmendia, C., (2002) for more information in lactobacillus strains and symptom improvement.
5. See Wilkins, T., & Sequoia, J. (2018) for more information on probiotics and inflammatory bowel disease.
6. See Underwood, M. (2022, February 6) for more information on B. infantis.
7. See Kunyeit, L. (2020) for more information on S. boulardii.
8. See Han, S., Lu, Y., Xie, J. (2019) for more information on probiotic transit time.

9. See Ciorba M. A. (2012) for more information on probiotics transit time.

10. See Fenster, K., Freeburg, B., (2019) for more information about the GI tract and probiotic colonization.

11. See Han, S., Lu, Y., Xie, J. (2019) for more information probiotic colonization.

12. See Cheng, J., & Ouwehand, A. C. (2020) for more information on acid reflux and probiotics.

13. See Ariola, J. (2018) for more information on collagen and gut health.

14. See Abrahams, M., O'Grady, R., & Prawitt, J. (2022) for more information on collagen and gut health.

15. See Perna, S., Alalwan, T. A. (2019) for more information on L-glutamine and gut health.

16. Gokulan, K., Kolluru, P. (2019). For more information on Aloe Vera and gut bacteria.

10. Natural Soothing Remedies for Digestive Symptoms

1. See Diez-Sampedro, A. (2019) for more information on gluten-free diets.

2. See National Center for Biotechnology Information (2022) for more information on Senna.

3. See Ohkusa, T., Koido (2019) for more information on probiotics and constipation.

4. See *8 Herbs To Benefit Gut Health*. (2022) for more information in herbal remedies and gut health

5. See *Milk thistle*. (n.d.). Mount Sinai Health System. (Retrieved September 15, 2022) for more information.

6. See *foodnavigator-usa.com. (2021, March 19)* for more information on nettle.

7. See Scazzocchio, B., Minghetti, L., & D'Archivio, M. (2020) for more information on gut health and turmeric.

11. What It Takes to Make Weight Loss Sustainable: A Gut-Health Centered Approach

1. See This Is What Happens To Your Body When You Crash Diet (2021) for more information on extreme diets and their effect on the human body.

Your Four-Week Gut Health Reset Plan

1. See Hadi, A., Pourmasoumi, M. (2021) for more information on the health benefits of apple cider vinegar.
2. See Abrahams, M., O'Grady, R., & Prawitt, J. (2022) for more information on collagen and gut health.
3. See Neyrinck, A. M., (2021) for more information on berberine and gut health.
4. See Chedid, V., Dhalla, S. (2014) for more information on SIBO and antimicrobial therapy.
5. See Center for Food Safety and Applied Nutrition. (2017) for more information on foods and gut diversity

REFERENCES

Abdominal Self-Massage. (n.d.). https://www.med.umich.edu/1libr/MBCP/AbdominalSelfmassage.pdf

Abrahams, M., O'Grady, R., & Prawitt, J. (2022). Effect of a Daily Collagen Peptide Supplement on Digestive Symptoms in Healthy Women: 2-Phase Mixed Methods Study. JMIR formative research, 6(5), e36339. https://doi.org/10.2196/36339

Achufusi, T., Sharma, A., Zamora, E. A., & Manocha, D. (2020). Small Intestinal Bacterial Overgrowth: Comprehensive Review of Diagnosis, Prevention, and Treatment Methods. *Cureus, 12*(6), e8860. https://doi.org/10.7759/cureus.8860

Akimbekov, N. S., Digel, I., Sherelkhan, D. K., Lutfor, A. B., & Razzaque, M. S. (2020). Vitamin D and the Host-Gut Microbiome: A Brief Overview. *Acta histochemica et cytochemica, 53*(3), 33–42. https://doi.org/10.1267/ahc.20011

An Increase in the Omega-6/Omega-3 Fatty Acid Ratio Increases the Risk for Obesity. *Nutrients, 8*(3), 128. https://doi.org/10.3390/nu8030128

Ansary, J., Forbes-Hernández, T. Y., Gil, E., Cianciosi, D., Zhang, J., Elexpuru-Zabaleta, M., Simal-Gandara, J., Giampieri, F., & Battino, M. (2020). Potential Health Benefit of Garlic Based on Human Intervention Studies: A Brief Overview. *Antioxidants (Basel, Switzerland), 9*(7), 619. https://doi.org/10.3390/antiox9070619

Appleton J. (2018). The Gut-Brain Axis: Influence of Microbiota on Mood and Mental Health. *Integrative medicine (Encinitas, Calif.), 17*(4), 28–32.

Al Kassa, I. (2016). Antiviral probiotics: A New Concept in Medical Sciences. New Insights on Antiviral Probiotics, 1–46. https://doi.org/10.1007/978-3-319-49688-7_1

Allonsius, C. N., Broek, M. F. L., de Boeck, I., Kiekens, S., Oerlemans, E. F. M., Kiekens, F., Foubert, K., Vandenheuvel, D., Cos, P., Delputte, P., & Lebeer, S. (2017). Interplay betweenLactobacillus rhamnosusGGandCandidaand the involvement of exopolysaccharides. Microbial Biotechnology, 10(6), 1753–1763. https://doi.org/10.1111/1751-7915.12799

Amen, D. G., MD. (2013). *Unleash the Power of the Female Brain.* Harmony/Rodale.

Ariola, J. (2018, November 5). *BENEFITS OF COLLAGEN FOR MAINTAINING A HEALTHY GUT.* Health Beat. https://www.flushinghospital.org/newsletter/benefits-of-collagen-for-maintaining-a-healthy-gut/

Arlinghaus, K. R., & Johnston, C. A. (2018). The Importance of Creating Habits and Routine. *American journal of lifestyle medicine, 13*(2), 142–144. https://doi.org/10.1177/1559827618818044

Aslam, H., Marx, W., Rocks, T., Loughman, A., Chandrasekaran, V., Ruusunen, A., Dawson, S. L., West, M., Mullarkey, E., Pasco, J. A., & Jacka, F. N. (2020). The effects of dairy and dairy derivatives on the gut micro-biota: a systematic literature review. *Gut microbes, 12*(1), 1799533. https://doi.org/10.1080/19490976.2020.1799533

Associated Diseases. (n.d.). SIBO - Small Intestine Bacterial Overgrowth. Retrieved September 13, 2022, from https://www.siboinfo.com/associated-diseases.html

Astrup, A., Teicholz, N., Magkos, F., Bier, D. M., Brenna, J. T., King, J. C., Mente, A., Ordovas, J. M., Volek, J. S., Yusuf, S., & Krauss, R. M. (2021). Dietary Saturated Fats and Health: Are the U.S. Guidelines Evidence-Based?. *Nutrients, 13*(10), 3305. https://doi.org/10.3390/nu13103305

Axe, D. J. C. (2018, March 21). *The 5 worst healthy sweeteners, and healthy alternatives.* Dr. Axe. https://draxe.com/nutrition/artificial-sweeteners/

Avena, N. M., Rada, P., & Hoebel, B. G. (2008). Evidence for sugar addiction: behavioral and neurochemical effects of intermittent, excessive sugar intake. *Neuroscience and biobehavioral reviews, 32*(1), 20–39. https://doi.org/10.1016/j.neubiorev.2007.04.019

Balali-Mood, M. (2021). *Toxic Mechanisms of Five Heavy Metals: Mercury, Lead, Chromium, Cadmium, and Arsenic.* Frontiers. https://www.frontiersin.org/articles/10.3389/fphar.2021.643972/full

Bellini, M., Tonarelli, S., Nagy, A. G., Pancetti, A., Costa, F., Ricchiuti, A., de Bortoli, N., Mosca, M., Marchi, S., & Rossi, A. (2020). Low FODMAP Diet: Evidence, Doubts, and Hopes. *Nutrients, 12*(1), 148. https://doi.org/10.3390/nu12010148

Bercik, P., Park, A. J., Sinclair, D., Khoshdel, A., Lu, J., Huang, X., Deng, Y., Blennerhassett, P. A., Fahnestock, M., Moine, D., Berger, B., Huizinga, J. D., Kunze, W., McLean, P. G., Bergonzelli, G. E., Collins, S. M., & Verdu, E. F. (2011). The anxiolytic effect of Bifidobacterium longum NCC3001 involves vagal pathways for gut-brain communication. *Neurogastroenterology and motility : the official journal of the European Gastrointestinal Motility Society, 23*(12), 1132–1139. https://doi.org/10.1111/j.1365-2982.2011.01796.x

Bertani, B., & Ruiz, N. (2018). Function and Biogenesis of Lipopolysaccha-rides. *EcoSal Plus, 8*(1), 10.1128/ecosalplus.ESP-0001-2018. https://doi.org/10.1128/ecosalplus.ESP-0001-2018

Bhandari P, Sapra A. (February 10, 2022) Low Fat Diet. [Updated 2022 Feb 10]. StatPearls, 1-5.https://www.ncbi.nlm.nih.gov/books/NBK553097/

Bian, X., Tu, P., Chi, L., Gao, B., Ru, H., & Lu, K. (2017). Saccharin induced liver inflammation in mice by altering the gut microbiota and its metabolic functions. Food and chemical toxicology : an international journal published for the British Industrial Biological Research Association, 107(Pt B), 530–539. https://doi.org/10.1016/j.fct.2017.04.045

Biswas, C. (2014, January 2). *Top 15 Glutamine-Rich Foods You Should Add To Your Diet*. STYLECRAZE. https://www.stylecraze.com/articles/glutamine-rich-foods-you-should-add-to-your-diet/

Breton, J., Massart, S., Vandamme, P., De Brandt, E., Pot, B., & Foligné, B. (2013). Ecotoxicology inside the gut: impact of heavy metals on the mouse microbiome. *BMC pharmacology & toxicology, 14*, 62. https://doi.org/10.1186/2050-6511-14-62

Bliss, E. S., & Whiteside, E. (2018). *The Gut-brain axis, the human gut mcrobiota and their integration in the development of obesity.* Frontiers in Physiology, 9. https://doi.org/10.3389/fphys.2018.00900

Blum, W., Zechmeister-Boltenstern, S., & Keiblinger, K. M. (2019). Does Soil Contribute to the Human Gut Microbiome?. *Microorganisms, 7*(9), 287. https://doi.org/10.3390/microorganisms7090287

Bundgaard-Nielsen, C., Knudsen, J., Leutscher, P., Lauritsen, M. B., Nyegaard, M., Hagstrøm, S., & Sørensen, S. (2020). Gut microbiota profiles of autism spectrum disorder and attention deficit/hyperactivity disorder: A systematic literature review. *Gut microbes, 11*(5), 1172–1187. https://doi.org/10.1080/19490976.2020.1748258

Buono, R., & Longo, V. D. (2019). When Fasting Gets Tough, the Tough Immune Cells Get Going—or Die. Cell, 178(5), 1038–1040. https://doi.org/10.1016/j.cell.2019.07.052

Camilleri, M. (2019). Leaky gut: mechanisms, measurement and clinical implications in humans. Gut, 68(8), 1516–1526. https://doi.org/10.1136/gutjnl-2019-318427

Caminero, A., Meisel, M., Jabri, B., & Verdu, E. F. (2019). Mechanisms by which gut microorganisms influence food sensitivities. *Nature reviews. Gastroenterology & hepatology, 16*(1), 7–18. https://doi.org/10.1038/s41575-018-0064-z

Carbone, J. W., & Pasiakos, S. M. (2019). Dietary Protein and Muscle Mass: Translating Science to Application and Health Benefit. *Nutrients, 11*(5), 1136. https://doi.org/10.3390/nu11051136

Caricilli, A. M., Castoldi, A., & Câmara, N. O. (2014). Intestinal barrier: A gentlemen's agreement between microbiota and immunity. World journal of gastrointestinal pathophysiology, 5(1), 18–32. https://doi.org/10.4291/wjgp.v5.i1.18

Center for Disease Control. (June 2021). Health Topics – Healthcare-associated Infections (HAI) https://www.cdc.gov/policy/polaris/healthtopics/hai/

index.html#:~:text=HAIs%20in%20U.S.%20hospitals%20have,early%20deaths%20and%20lost%20productivity.

Center for Food Safety and Applied Nutrition. (2017, December 7). *FDA Completes Review of Qualified Health Claim Petition for Macadamia Nuts and the Risk of Coronary Heart Disease*. U.S. Food and Drug Administration. https://www.fda.gov/food/cfsan-constituent-updates/fda-completes-review-qualified-health-claim-petition-macadamia-nuts-and-risk-coronary-heart-disease.

Chedid, V., Dhalla, S., Clarke, J. O., Roland, B. C., Dunbar, K. B., Koh, J., Justino, E., Tomakin, E., & Mullin, G. E. (2014). Herbal therapy is equivalent to rifaximin for the treatment of small intestinal bacterial overgrowth. *Global advances in health and medicine, 3*(3), 16–24. https://doi.org/10.7453/gahmj.2014.019

Cheng, J., & Ouwehand, A. C. (2020). Gastroesophageal Reflux Disease and Probiotics: A Systematic Review. *Nutrients, 12*(1), 132. https://doi.org/10.3390/nu12010132

Ciorba M. A. (2012). A gastroenterologist's guide to probiotics. *Clinical gastroenterology and hepatology : the official clinical practice journal of the American Gastroenterological Association, 10*(9), 960–968. https://doi.org/10.1016/j.cgh.2012.03.024

Clark, A. (2020, March 11). *Protein consumption, the gut microbiota and health*. Gut Microbiota for Health. https://www.gutmicrobiotaforhealth.com/protein-consumption-the-gut-microbiota-and-health/

Collier R. (2013). Intermittent fasting: the science of going without. *CMAJ : Canadian Medical Association journal = journal de l'Association medicale canadienne, 185*(9), E363–E364. https://doi.org/10.1503/cmaj.109-4451

Colonoscopy - Everything you need to know about the procedure. (n.d.). Retrieved September 9, 2022, from https://www.mymed.com/tests-procedures/colonoscopy

Cruzat, V., Macedo Rogero, M., Noel Keane, K., Curi, R., & Newsholme, P. (2018). Glutamine: Metabolism and Immune Function, Supplementation and Clinical Translation. *Nutrients, 10*(11), 1564. https://doi.org/10.3390/nu10111564

Cuthbert, S. C., & Goodheart, G. J. (2007, March 6). On the reliability and validity of manual muscle testing: a literature review. *Chiropractic &Amp; Osteopathy, 15*(1). https://doi.org/10.1186/1746-1340-15-4

Daley, C. A., Abbott, A., Doyle, P. S., Nader, G. A., & Larson, S. (2010). A review of fatty acid profiles and antioxidant content in grass-fed and grain-fed beef. *Nutrition journal, 9*, 10. https://doi.org/10.1186/1475-2891-9-10

Dang, A. T., & Marsland, B. J. (2019). Microbes, metabolites, and the gut–lung axis. Mucosal Immunology, 12(4), 843–850. https://doi.org/10.1038/s41385-019-0160-6

de Oliveira Santos, G. C., Vasconcelos, C. C., Lopes, A. J. O., de Sousa Cartágenes, M. D. S., Filho, A. K. D. B., do Nascimento, F. R. F., Ramos, R. M., Pires, E. R. R. B., de Andrade, M. S., Rocha, F. M. G., & de Andrade Monteiro, C. (2018a). Candida Infections and Therapeutic Strategies: Mechanisms of Action for Traditional and Alternative Agents. Frontiers in Microbiology, 9. https://doi.org/10.3389/fmicb.2018.01351

Derrien, M., & van Hylckama Vlieg, J. E. (2015, June). Fate, activity, and impact of ingested bacteria within the human gut microbiota. *Trends in Microbiology*, *23*(6), 354–366. https://doi.org/10.1016/j.tim.2015.03.002

Diabetes. (2021, November 10). World Health Organization. https://www.who.int/news-room/fact-sheets/detail/diabetes

Diez-Sampedro, A., Olenick, M., Maltseva, T., & Flowers, M. (2019). A Gluten-Free Diet, Not an Appropriate Choice without a Medical Diagnosis. *Journal of nutrition and metabolism*, *2019*, 2438934. https://doi.org/10.1155/2019/2438934

Diether, N., & Willing, B. (2019). Microbial Fermentation of Dietary Protein: An Important Factor in Diet–Microbe–Host Interaction. *Microorganisms*, *7*(1), 19. MDPI AG. Retrieved from http://dx.doi.org/10.3390/microorganisms7010019

The difference between celiac disease and gluten intolerance. (2018). Closing the Gap Healthcare. https://www.closingthegap.ca/the-difference-between-celiac-disease-gluten-intolerance-and-wheat-allergy/

Division of Foodborne, Waterborne, and Environmental Diseases | CDC. (n.d.). Center for Disease Control: Facts About Candida. https://www.cdc.gov/ncezid/dfwed/index.html\

DiNicolantonio, J. J., & O'Keefe, J. H. (2017). Good Fats versus Bad Fats: A Comparison of Fatty Acids in the Promotion of Insulin Resistance, Inflammation, and Obesity. *Missouri medicine*, *114*(4), 303–307

DiNicolantonio, J. J., O'Keefe, J. H., & Wilson, W. (2018). Subclinical magnesium deficiency: a principal driver of cardiovascular disease and a public health crisis. *Open heart*, *5*(1), e000668. https://doi.org/10.1136/openhrt-2017-000668

Drago, S., El Asmar, R., Di Pierro, M., Grazia Clemente, M., Tripathi, A., Sapone, A., Thakar, M., Iacono, G., Carroccio, A., D'Agate, C., Not, T., Zampini, L., Catassi, C., & Fasano, A. (2006). Gliadin, zonulin and gut permeability: Effects on celiac and non-celiac intestinal mucosa and intestinal cell lines. *Scandinavian journal of gastroenterology*, *41*(4), 408–419. https://doi.org/10.1080/00365520500235334

Dyerberg, J., Madsen, P., Møller, J., Aardestrup, I., & Schmidt, E. (2010). Bioavailability of marine n-3 fatty acid formulations. *Prostaglandins, Leukotrienes and Essential Fatty Acids, 83*(3), 137–141. https://doi.org/10.1016/j.plefa.2010.06.007

Eight Herbs To Benefit Gut Health. (2022). Mountain Mel's. https://www.mountainmels.com/blogs/news/supporting-gut-health#:%7E:text=Calendula%20can%20improve%20digestion%20and,heal%20your%20damaged%20gut%20wall!

Eleven Safest Non-Toxic Cookware Brands For A Healthy Kitchen in 2022. (n.d.). Sustainable Kind Living. Retrieved October 20, 2022, from https://sustainablykindliving.com/non-toxic-cookware/

Ellis, J. L., Karl, J. P., Oliverio, A. M., Fu, X., Soares, J. W., Wolfe, B. E., Hernandez, C. J., Mason, J. B., & Booth, S. L. (2021). Dietary vitamin K is remodeled by gut microbiota and influences community composition. *Gut microbes, 13*(1), 1–16. https://doi.org/10.1080/19490976.2021.1887721

Endoscopy. (2022, August 22). Merck Manuals Consumer Version. Retrieved September 9, 2022, from https://www.merckmanuals.com/home/digestive-disorders/diagnosis-of-digestive-disorders/endoscopy

Fajstova, A., Galanova, N., Coufal, S., Malkova, J., Kostovcik, M., Cermakova, M., Pelantova, H., Kuzma, M., Sediva, B., Hudcovic, T., Hrncir, T., Tlaskalova-Hogenova, H., Kverka, M., & Kostovcikova, K. (2020). Diet Rich in Simple Sugars Promotes Pro-Inflammatory Response via Gut Microbiota Alteration and TLR4 Signaling. *Cells, 9*(12), 2701. https://doi.org/10.3390/cells9122701

Fasano A. (2012). Intestinal permeability and its regulation by zonulin: diagnostic and therapeutic implications. *Clinical gastroenterology and hepatology : the official clinical practice journal of the American Gastroenterological Association, 10*(10), 1096–1100. https://doi.org/10.1016/j.cgh.2012.08.012

Fenster, K., Freeburg, B., Hollard, C., Wong, C., Rønhave Laursen, R., & Ouwehand, A. C. (2019). The Production and Delivery of Probiotics: A Review of a Practical Approach. *Microorganisms, 7*(3), 83. https://doi.org/10.3390/microorganisms7030083

The Five Things People Regret Most On Their Deathbed. (2013, December 6). Business Insider. https://www.businessinsider.com/5-things-people-regret-on-their-deathbed-2013-12?international=true&r=US&IR=T

FODMAP Diet: What You Need to Know. (2021, December 29). Johns Hopkins Medicine. https://www.hopkinsmedicine.org/health/wellness-and-prevention/fodmap-diet-what-you-need-to-know#:%7E:text=What%20is%20FODMAP%3F,digestive%20distress%20after%20eating%20them.

Food Allergy Diagnosis and Testing. (n.d.). FoodAllergy.org. Retrieved September 7, 2022, from https://www.foodallergy.org/research-innovation/accelerating-innovation/food-allergy-diagnosis-and-testing

Foodnavigator-usa.com. (2021, March 19). *Research explores potential of nettle as a functional food*. Retrieved September 15, 2022, from https://www.foodnavi gator-usa.com/Article/2021/03/19/Research-explores-potential-of-nettle-as-a-functional-food#

Forgiveness: Your Health Depends on It. (2021, November 1). Johns Hopkins Medicine. https://www.hopkinsmedicine.org/health/wellness-and-preven tion/forgiveness-your-health-depends-on-it

Franchi, F., Yaranov, D. M., Rollini, F., Rivas, A., Rivas Rios, J., Been, L., Tani, Y., Tokuda, M., Iida, T., Hayashi, N., Angiolillo, D. J., & Mooradian, A. D. (2021). Effects of D-allulose on glucose tolerance and insulin response to a standard oral sucrose load: results of a prospective, randomized, crossover study. BMJ Open Diabetes Research & Care, 9(1), e001939. https://doi.org/10.1136/bmjdrc-2020-001939

Frederick Health. (2021, July 29). 10 signs of an unhealthy gut. Frederick Health. Retrieved April 22, 2022, from https://www.frederickhealth.org/news/2021/july/10-signs-of-an-unhealthy-gut/

Furman, D., Campisi, J., Verdin, E., Carrera-Bastos, P., Targ, S., Franceschi, C., Ferrucci, L., Gilroy, D. W., Fasano, A., Miller, G. W., Miller, A. H., Manto-vani, A., Weyand, C. M., Barzilai, N., Goronzy, J. J., Rando, T. A., Effros, R. B., Lucia, A., Kleinstreuer, N., & Slavich, G. M. (2019). Chronic inflamma-tion in the etiology of disease across the life span. *Nature medicine, 25*(12), 1822–1832. https://doi.org/10.1038/s41591-019-0675-0

Gaon, D., Garmendia, C., Murrielo, N. O., de Cucco Games, A., Cerchio, A., Quintas, R., González, S. N., & Oliver, G. (2002). Effect of Lactobacillus strains (L. casei and L. Acidophillus Strains cerela) on bacterial over-growth-related chronic diarrhea. *Medicina, 62*(2), 159–163.

Gaci, N., Borrel, G., Tottey, W., O'Toole, P. W., & Brugère, J. F. (2014). Archaea and the human gut: new beginning of an old story. *World journal of gastroenterology, 20*(43), 16062–16078. https://doi.org/10.3748/wjg.v20.i43.16062

Gene Food. https://www.mygenefood.com/blog/which-probiotic-strains-get-rid-of-candida/

Ginsberg H. N. (2000). Insulin resistance and cardiovascular disease. The Journal of clinical investigation, 106(4), 453–458. https://doi.org/10.1172/JCI10762

Glenny, E. M., Bulik-Sullivan, E. C., Tang, Q., Bulik, C. M., & Carroll, I. M. (2017, July 5). Eating Disorders and the Intestinal Microbiota: Mechanisms of Energy Homeostasis and Behavioral Influence. *Current Psychiatry Reports, 19*(8). https://doi.org/10.1007/s11920-017-0797-3

Ghoshal, U. C., Shukla, R., & Ghoshal, U. (2017, March 15). Small Intestinal Bacterial Overgrowth and Irritable Bowel Syndrome: A Bridge between

Functional Organic Dichotomy. *Gut And Liver*, *11*(2), 196–208. https://doi.org/10.5009/gnl16126

Gokulan, K., Kolluru, P., Cerniglia, C. E., & Khare, S. (2019). Dose-Dependent Effects of Aloin on the Intestinal Bacterial Community Structure, Short Chain Fatty Acids Metabolism and Intestinal Epithelial Cell Permeability. *Frontiers in microbiology*, *10*, 474. https://doi.org/10.3389/fmicb.2019.00474

The Gut Healing Ninja. (2021). Heavy Metal Exposure and Gut Health. https://www.theguthealingninja.com/blog/heavy-metals-gut-health

The Gut Healing Ninja. (2021). *4 Steps to Healing Food Sensitivities*. https://www.theguthealingninja.com/blog/healing-food-sensitivities

Hadi, A., Pourmasoumi, M., Najafgholizadeh, A., Clark, C. C. T., & Esmail-lzadeh, A. (2021). The effect of apple cider vinegar on lipid profiles and glycemic parameters: a systematic review and meta-analysis of randomized clinical trials. *BMC complementary medicine and therapies*, *21*(1), 179. https://doi.org/10.1186/s12906-021-03351-w

Han, Y., Zhang, L., Liu, X. Q., Zhao, Z. J., & Lv, L. X. (2017). Effect of glucomannan on functional constipation in children: a systematic review and meta-analysis of randomised controlled trials. *Asia Pacific journal of clinical nutrition*, *26*(3), 471–477. https://doi.org/10.6133/apjcn.032016.03

Han, S., Lu, Y., Xie, J., Fei, Y., Zheng, G., Wang, Z., Liu, J., Lv, L., Ling, Z., Berglund, B., Yao, M., & Li, L. (2021, March 10). Probiotic Gastrointestinal Transit and Colonization After Oral Administration: A Long Journey. *Frontiers in Cellular and Infection Microbiology*, *11*. https://doi.org/10.3389/fcimb.2021.609722

Harris, L. (2021, October 13). *10 Simple Ways to Avoid Microplastics in Your Everyday Life*. EcoWatch. https://www.ecowatch.com/avoid-microplastics-at-home-2655282616.html

Harvard Health. (2016, October 14). Can gut bacteria improve your health? https://www.health.harvard.edu/staying-healthy/can-gut-bacteria-improve-your-health

Harvard Health. (2016a, June 16). Loneliness has same risk as smoking for heart disease. Retrieved October 21, 2022, from https://www.health.harvard.edu/staying-healthy/loneliness-has-same-risk-as-smoking-for-heart-disease

Hatakka, K., Ahola, A., Yli-Knuuttila, H., Richardson, M., Poussa, T., Meurman, J., & Korpela, R. (2007). Probiotics Reduce the Prevalence of Oral Candida in the Elderly—a Randomized Controlled Trial. Journal of Dental Research, *86*(2), 125–130. https://doi.org/10.1177/154405910708600204

Hijikata, Y., & Yamada, S. (2011). Walking just after a meal seems to be more effective for weight loss than waiting for one hour to walk after a meal. *International journal of general medicine, 4,* 447–450. https://doi.org/10.2147/IJGM.S18837

Heavy Metals | The Caribbean Environment Programme (CEP). (2008). Caribbean Environment Programme. https://www.unep.org/cep/heavy-metals#:%7E:text=Heavy%20metals%20normally%20occur%20in,which%20can%20pollute%20the%20environment

Head K. A. (2008). Natural approaches to prevention and treatment of infections of the lower urinary tract. *Alternative medicine review : a journal of clinical therapeutic, 13*(3), 227–244.

Histamine Intolerance Awareness. (2020, May 4). *The Food List.* Histamine Intolerance. https://www.histamineintolerance.org.uk/about/the-food-diary/the-food-list/

History of the Dietary Guidelines | Dietary Guidelines for Americans. (2020). USDA Website. https://www.dietaryguidelines.gov/about-dietary-guidelines/history-dietary-guidelines

Hollon, J., Puppa, E. L., Greenwald, B., Goldberg, E., Guerrerio, A., & Fasano, A. (2015). Effect of gliadin on permeability of intestinal biopsy explants from celiac disease patients and patients with non-celiac gluten sensitivity. *Nutrients, 7*(3), 1565–1576 https://doi.org/10.3390/nu7031565

Hooper, L., Martin, N., Jimoh, O. F., Kirk, C., Foster, E., & Abdelhamid, A. S. (2020). Reduction in saturated fat intake for cardiovascular disease. *The Cochrane database of systematic reviews, 8*(8), CD011737. https://doi.org/10.1002/14651858.CD011737.pub3

How Do Thoughts and Emotions Affect Health? (2016). Taking Charge of Your Health & Wellbeing. https://www.takingcharge.csh.umn.edu/how-do-thoughts-and-emotions-affect-health

Househam, A. M., Peterson, C. T., Mills, P. J., & Chopra, D. (2017). The Effects of Stress and Meditation on the Immune System, Human Microbiota, and Epigenetics. *Advances in mind-body medicine, 31*(4), 10–25

Huang Z, Weng Y, Shen Q, Zhao Y, Jin Y. Microplastic: A potential threat to human and animal health by interfering with the intestinal barrier function and changing the intestinal microenvironment. Sci Total Environ. 2021 Sep 1;785:147365. doi: 10.1016/j.scitotenv.2021.147365. Epub 2021 Apr 27. PMID: 33933760

Huh, J. (2022, May 20). *What Is Hydrogen Sulfide SIBO and How Is It Treated?* Dr. Michael Ruscio, DNM, DC. Retrieved September 13, 2022, from https://drruscio.com/hydrogen-sulfide-sibo/

Hypochlorhydria (Low Stomach Acid): Symptoms, Tests, Treatment. (n.d.). Cleveland Clinic. https://my.clevelandclinic.org/health/diseases/23392-hypochlorhydria

Irritable bowel syndrome - Diagnosis and treatment - Mayo Clinic. (2021,

December 1). . Retrieved September 12, 2022, from https://www.mayoclinic.org/diseases-conditions/irritable-bowel-syndrome/diagnosis-treatment/drc-20360064

Jackson, E., Shoemaker, R., Larian, N., & Cassis, L. (2017). Adipose Tissue as a Site of Toxin Accumulation. Comprehensive Physiology, 1085–1135. https://doi.org/10.1002/cphy.c160038

Jariwalla RJ, Lalezari J, Cenko D, Mansour SE, Kumar A, Gangapurkar B, Nakamura D. Restoration of blood total glutathione status and lymphocyte function following alpha-lipoic acid supplementation in patients with HIV infection. J Altern Complement Med. 2008 Mar;14(2):139-46. doi: 10.1089/acm.2006.6397. PMID: 18315507.

Jiang, Z., Sun, Ty., He, Y. *et al.* Dietary fruit and vegetable intake, gut microbiota, and type 2 diabetes: results from two large human cohort studies. *BMC Med* 18, 371 (2020). https://doi.org/10.1186/s12916-020-01842-0

Kelly J. D., 4th (2019). Your Best Life: Managing Negative Thoughts-The Choice is Yours. *Clinical orthopaedics and related research*, 477(6), 1291–1293. https://doi.org/10.1097/CORR.0000000000000791

Kelly, J. R., Kennedy, P. J., Cryan, J. F., Dinan, T. G., Clarke, G., & Hyland, N. P. (2015). Breaking down the barriers: the gut microbiome, intestinal permeability and stress-related psychiatric disorders. Frontiers in Cellular Neuroscience, 9. https://doi.org/10.3389/fncel.2015.00392

Khalili H. (2016). Risk of Inflammatory Bowel Disease with Oral Contraceptives and Menopausal Hormone Therapy: Current Evidence and Future Directions. *Drug safety*, 39(3), 193–197. https://doi.org/10.1007/s40264-015-0372-y

Kim, D. B., Paik, C. N., Song, D. S., Kim, Y. J., & Lee, J. M. (2018, March 22). The characteristics of small intestinal bacterial overgrowth in patients with gallstone diseases. *Journal of Gastroenterology and Hepatology*, 33(8), 1477–1484. https://doi.org/10.1111/jgh.14113

Kinney, J. W., Bemiller, S. M., Murtishaw, A. S., Leisgang, A. M., Salazar, A. M., & Lamb, B. T. (2018). Inflammation as a central mechanism in Alzheimer's disease. Alzheimer's & Dementia: Translational Research & Clinical Interventions, 4(1), 575–590. https://doi.org/10.1016/j.trci.2018.06.014

Klintberg, B., Berglund, N., Lilja, G., Wickman, M., & van Hage-Hamsten, M. (2001). Fewer allergic respiratory disorders among farmers' children in a closed birth cohort from Sweden. *The European respiratory journal*, 17(6), 1151–1157. https://doi.org/10.1183/09031936.01.00027301

Krishna Rao, R. (2012). Role of Glutamine in Protection of Intestinal Epithelial Tight Junctions. Journal of Epithelial Biology and Pharmacology, 5(1), 47–54. https://doi.org/10.2174/1875044301205010047

Kumamoto, C. A. (2011). Inflammation and gastrointestinal Candida colonization. Current Opinion in Microbiology, 14(4), 386–391. https://doi.org/10.1016/j.mib.2011.07.015

Kunyeit, L., K A, A. A., & Rao, R. P. (2020). Application of Probiotic Yeasts on *Candida* Species Associated Infection. *Journal of fungi (Basel, Switzerland), 6*(4), 189. https://doi.org/10.3390/jof6040189

La Berge, A. F. (2007). How the Ideology of Low Fat Conquered America. *Journal of the History of Medicine and Allied Sciences, 63*(2), 139–177. https://doi.org/10.1093/jhmas/jrn001

Lane, A., Dalkie, N., Henderson, L., Irwin, J., & Rostami, K. (2021). An elemental diet is effective in the management of diversion colitis. *Gastroenterology and hepatology from bed to bench, 14*(1), 81–84.

Laxative Use: What to Know. (2019). Cornell Health. https://health.cornell.edu

Lee, D. Y. (n.d.). Vitamin and mineral deficiencies in inflammatory bowel disease. *Up to Date.*

Levy, J. C. (2019, April 25). What Is Candida Die Off? 6 Ways to Manage Symptoms. Dr. Axe. https://draxe.com/health/candida-die-off/

Lew, L. C., Hor, Y. Y., Yusoff, N., Choi, S. B., Yusoff, M., Roslan, N. S., Ahmad, A., Mohammad, J., Abdullah, M., Zakaria, N., Wahid, N., Sun, Z., Kwok, L. Y., Zhang, H., & Liong, M. T. (2019). Probiotic Lactobacillus plantarum P8 alleviated stress and anxiety while enhancing memory and cognition in stressed adults: A randomised, double-blind, placebo-controlled study. Clinical nutrition (Edinburgh, Scotland), 38(5), 2053–2064. https://doi.org/10.1016/j.clnu.2018.09.010

Lewis, S. J., & Heaton, K. W. (1997, January). Stool Form Scale as a Useful Guide to Intestinal Transit Time. *Scandinavian Journal of Gastroenterology, 32*(9), 920–924. https://doi.org/10.3109/00365529709011203

Li, Q., Chang, Y., Zhang, K., Chen, H., Tao, S., & Zhang, Z. (2020). Implication of the gut microbiome composition of type 2 diabetic patients from northern China. Scientific Reports, 10(1). https://doi.org/10.1038/s41598-020-62224-

Li, Y., Hao, Y., Fan, F., & Zhang, B. (2018). The Role of Microbiome in Insomnia, Circadian Disturbance and Depression. Frontiers in Psychiatry, 9. https://doi.org/10.3389/fpsyt.2018.00669

Liu, T., Liang, X., Lei, C., Huang, Q., Song, W., Fang, R., Li, C., Li, X., Mo, H., Sun, N., Lv, H., & Liu, Z. (2020). High-Fat Diet Affects Heavy Metal Accumulation and Toxicity to Mice Liver and Kidney Probably via Gut Microbiota. *Frontiers in Microbiology, 11*. https://doi.org/10.3389/fmicb.2020.01604

Lopresti, A. L., Smith, S. J., Rea, A., & Michel, S. (2021). Efficacy of a curcumin extract (Curcugen™) on gastrointestinal symptoms and intestinal microbiota in adults with self-reported digestive complaints: a randomised, double-blind, placebo-controlled study. *BMC complementary medicine and therapies, 21*(1), 40. https://doi.org/10.1186/s12906-021-03220-6

Losso JN. Food Processing, Dysbiosis, Gastrointestinal Inflammatory Diseases, and Antiangiogenic Functional Foods or Beverages. Annu Rev Food Sci Technol. 2021 Mar 25;12:235-258. doi: 10.1146/annurev-food-062520-090235. Epub 2021 Jan 19. PMID: 33467906.

Lotta, L. A., Abbasi, A., Sharp, S. J., Sahlqvist, A. S., Waterworth, D., Brosnan, J. M., Scott, R. A., Langenberg, C., & Wareham, N. J. (2015). Definitions of Metabolic Health and Risk of Future Type 2 Diabetes in BMI Categories: A Systematic Review and Network Meta-analysis. Diabetes care, 38(11), 2177–2187. https://doi.org/10.2337/dc15-1218

Ma, T., Jin, H., Kwok, L. Y., Sun, Z., Liong, M. T., & Zhang, H. (2021). Probiotic consumption relieved human stress and anxiety symptoms possibly via modulating the neuroactive potential of the gut microbiota. Neurobiology of stress, 14, 100294. https://doi.org/10.1016/j.ynstr.2021.100294

Madison, A., & Kiecolt-Glaser, J. K. (2019). Stress, depression, diet, and the gut microbiota: human-bacteria interactions at the core of psychoneuroimmunology and nutrition. *Current opinion in behavioral sciences, 28,* 105–110. https://doi.org/10.1016/j.cobeha.2019.01.011

Martins, N., Ferreira, I. C., Barros, L., Silva, S., & Henriques, M. (2014). Candidiasis: predisposing factors, prevention, diagnosis and alternative treatment. *Mycopathologia, 177*(5-6), 223–240. https://doi.org/10.1007/s11046-014-9749-1

Matthew BSc, PhD, M. J. (2014). Part 1: The Human Gut Microbiome in Health and Disease. Integrative medicine. Integrative Medicine: A Clinician's Journal, 13(6), 17–22.

Matthews, H. L. B. A. (2021, June 28). Which Probiotic Strains Inhibit Candida?

Mayo Clinic. Stress management (2021)https://www.mayoclinic.org/healthy-lifestyle/stress-management/in-depth/stress/art-20046037#:~:text=Adrenaline%20increases%20your%20heart%20rate,of%20substances%20that%20repair%20tissues.

Meroni, M., Longo, M., & Dongiovanni, P. (2019). Alcohol or Gut Microbiota: Who Is the Guilty?. *International journal of molecular sciences*

Miller, A. L., Bessho, S., Grando, K., & Tükel, Ç. (2021). Microbiome or Infections: Amyloid-Containing Biofilms as a Trigger for Complex Human Diseases. *Frontiers in immunology, 12,* 638867. https://doi.org/10.3389/fimmu.2021.638867

Milk thistle. (n.d.). Mount Sinai Health System. Retrieved September 15, 2022, from https://www.mountsinai.org/health-library/herb/milk-thistle#:%7E:

text=Several%20scientific%20studies%20suggest%20that,antioxi-dant%20and%20anti%2Dinflammatory%20properties.

Mohr, A. E., Gumpricht, E., Sears, D. D., & Sweazea, K. L. (2021). Recent advances and health implications of dietary fasting regimens on the gut microbiome. *American journal of physiology. Gastrointestinal and liver physiology, 320*(5), G847–G863. https://doi.org/10.1152/ajpgi.00475.2020

Monda, V., Villano, I., Messina, A., Valenzano, A., Esposito, T., Moscatelli, F., Viggiano, A., Cibelli, G., Chieffi, S., Monda, M., & Messina, G. (2017). Exercise Modifies the Gut Microbiota with Positive Health Effects. *Oxidative medicine and cellular longevity, 2017*, 3831972. https://doi.org/10.1155/2017/3831972

Morowitz, M. J., Carlisle, E. M., & Alverdy, J. C. (2011). Contributions of intestinal bacteria to nutrition and metabolism in the critically ill. *The Surgical clinics of North America, 91*(4), 771–viii. https://doi.org/10.1016/j.suc.2011.05.001

Moskowitz, R. (2020, November 3). *Micronutrients: Why They're Important for Gut Health and How to Get Enough of Them.* ModifyHealth. Retrieved September 14, 2022, from https://modifyhealth.com/blogs/blog/micronutrients-why-they-re-important-for-gut-health-and-how-to-get-enough-of-them

Mullins, A. P., & Arjmandi, B. H. (2021). Health Benefits of Plant-Based Nutrition: Focus on Beans in Cardiometabolic Diseases. *Nutrients, 13*(2), 519. https://doi.org/10.3390/nu13020519

Naleway A. L. (2004). Asthma and atopy in rural children: is farming protective?. *Clinical medicine & research, 2*(1), 5–12. https://doi.org/10.3121/cmr.2.1.5

National Center for Biotechnology Information (2022). PubChem Compound Summary for CID 5199, Sennosides. Retrieved July 21, 2022 from https://pubchem.ncbi.nlm.nih.gov/compound/SennosidesNeyrinck, A. M., Sánchez, C. R., Rodriguez, J., Cani, P. D., Bindels, L. B., & Delzenne, N. M. (2021). Prebiotic Effect of Berberine and Curcumin Is Associated with the Improvement of Obesity in Mice. Nutrients, 13(5), 1436. https://doi.org/10.3390/nu13051436

Navarro-Tapia, E., Almeida-Toledano, L., Sebastiani, G., Serra-Delgado, M., García-Algar, S., & Andreu-Fernández, V. (2021). Effects of Microbiota Imbalance in Anxiety and Eating Disorders: Probiotics as Novel Therapeutic Approaches. International Journal of Molecular Sciences, 22(5), 2351. https://doi.org/10.3390/ijms22052351

Nestle, M. (2018, October 23). *Superfoods' Origins in Marketing and Industry Research.* The Atlantic. https://www.theatlantic.com/health/archive/2018/10/superfoods-marketing-ploy/573583/

Neu, J., & Rushing, J. (2011). Cesarean Versus Vaginal Delivery: Long-term

Infant Outcomes and the Hygiene Hypothesis. Clinics in Perinatology, 38(2), 321–331. https://doi.org/10.1016/j.clp.2011.03.008

The Neurobiology of Substance Use, Misuse, and Addiction | Surgeon General's Report on Alcohol, Drugs, and Health. (2016). SurgeonGeneral.Gov. https://addiction.surgeongeneral.gov/executive-summary/report/neurobi ology-substance-use-misuse-and-addiction

Ngkelo, A. (2012, January 12). LPS induced inflammatory responses in human peripheral blood mononuclear cells is mediated through NOX4 and Giα dependent PI-3kinase signalling - Journal of Inflammation. BioMed Central. Retrieved September 14, 2022, from https://journal-inflammation. biomedcentral.com/articles/10.1186/1476-9255-9-1

Nguyen, J. (2021, June 22). Probiotics Can Reduce Stress and Improve Mood. Here's Why. Gene Food. https://www.mygenefood.com/blog/probiotics-reduce-stress-improve-mood/

Nutrition, G. B. (2020, August 19). *Why fats matter to your gut and general health.* Gutsy By Nutrition | Health & Wellness. https://gutsybynutrition.com.au/ gutsy-by-nutrition-blog/2020/8/18/why-fats-matter-to-your-gut-and-general-health

Obesity and overweight. (2021, June 9). The World Health Organization. https://www.who.int/news-room/fact-sheets/detail/obesity-and-over weight#:%7E:text=In%202016%2C%20more%20than%201.9,kills%20-more%20people%20than%20underweight.

Office of Dietary Supplements - Omega-3 Fatty Acids. (2022, June 2). National Institute of Health. https://ods.od.nih.gov/factsheets/Omega3FattyAcids-HealthProfessional/

Ohkusa, T., Koido, S., Nishikawa, Y., & Sato, N. (2019). Gut Microbiota and Chronic Constipation: A Review and Update. *Frontiers in medicine, 6,* 19. https://doi.org/10.3389/fmed.2019.00019

Olaimat, A. N., Aolymat, I., Al-Holy, M., Ayyash, M., Abu Ghoush, M., Al-Nabulsi, A. A., Osaili, T., Apostolopoulos, V., Liu, S. Q., & Shah, N. P. (2020). The potential application of probiotics and prebiotics for the prevention and treatment of COVID-19. Npj Science of Food, 4(1). https:// doi.org/10.1038/s41538-020-00078-9

Ordovas, J. M., Ferguson, L. R., Tai, E. S., & Mathers, J. C. (2018). Personalised nutrition and health. *BMJ (Clinical research ed.), 361,* bmj.k2173. https://doi. org/10.1136/bmj.k2173

Paddock, C., PhD. (2018, August 8). Could probiotics cause "brain fog" and bloating? Medical News Today. https://www.medicalnewstoday.com/arti cles/322712#Beware-of-excessive-use-of- probiotics

Panacer, K., Whorwell, P. J. (2019). Dietary Lectin exclusion: The next big food trend?. *World journal of gastroenterology, 25*(24), 2973–2976. https://doi.org/10.3748/wjg.v25.i24.2973

Patterson, R. E., Laughlin, G. A., LaCroix, A. Z., Hartman, S. J., Natarajan, L., Senger, C. M., Martínez, M. E., Villaseñor, A., Sears, D. D., Marinac, C. R., & Gallo, L. C. (2015). Intermittent Fasting and Human Metabolic Health. *Journal of the Academy of Nutrition and Dietetics, 115*(8), 1203–1212. https://doi.org/10.1016/j.jand.2015.02.018

Perna, S., Alalwan, T. A., Alaali, Z., Alnashaba, T., Gasparri, C., Infantino, V., Hammad, L., Riva, A., Petrangolini, G., Allegrini, P., & Rondanelli, M. (2019). The Role of Glutamine in the Complex Interaction between Gut Microbiota and Health: A Narrative Review. *International journal of molecular sciences, 20*(20), 5232. https://doi.org/10.3390/ijms20205232

Petersen, C., & Round, J. L. (2014). Defining dysbiosis and its influence on host immunity and disease. Cellular Microbiology, 16(7), 1024–1033. https://doi.org/10.1111/cmi.12308

Rahimzadeh, R.i, M., Kazemi, S., & Moghadamnia, A. A. (2017). Cadmium toxicity and treatment: An update. *Caspian journal of internal medicine, 8*(3), 135–145. https://doi.org/10.22088/cjim.8.3.135

Rakul, D. (2018). The Elimination Diet (4th ed.). Elsevier, Inc.

Rao, S., Tan, G., Abdulla, H., Yu, S., Larion, S., & Leelasinjaroen, P. (2018). Does colectomy predispose to small intestinal bacterial (SIBO) and fungal overgrowth (SIFO)?. *Clinical and translational gastroenterology, 9*(4), 146. https://doi.org/10.1038/s41424-018-0011-x

Reynolds, A. N., & Venn, B. J. (2018). The Timing of Activity after Eating Affects the Glycaemic Response of Healthy Adults: A Randomised Controlled Trial. Nutrients, 10(11), 1743. https://doi.org/10.3390/nu10111743

An RD Explains How Blood Sugar Affects Food Cravings. (2020, July 18). HUM Nutrition Blog. https://www.humnutrition.com/blog/how-blood-sugar-affects-food-cravings/

Rifaximin (Oral Route). (2022, February 14). Â . Retrieved September 9, 2022, from https://www.mayoclinic.org/drugs-supplements/rifaximin-oral-route/side-effects/drg-20065817

Rinninella, E., Cintoni, M., Raoul, P., Lopetuso, L. R., Scaldaferri, F., Pulcini, G., Miggiano, G., Gasbarrini, A., & Mele, M. C. (2019). Food Components and Dietary Habits: Keys for a Healthy Gut Microbiota Composition. *Nutrients, 11*(10), 2393. https://doi.org/10.3390/nu11102393

Roberts, M. (2020, February 18). *FOUR Tactics to Improve Bile Flow*. Advanced Naturopathic. Retrieved September 12, 2022, from https://advancednaturopathic.com/four-tactics-to-improve-bile-flow/

Rossoni, R. D., de Barros, P. P., de Alvarenga, J. A., Ribeiro, F. D. C., Velloso, M. D. S.,

Fuchs, B. B., Mylonakis, E., Jorge, A. O. C., & Junqueira, J. C. (2018). Antifungal activity of clinical Lactobacillus strains against Candida albicans biofilms: identification of potential probiotic candidates to prevent oral candidiasis. Biofouling, 34(2), 212–225. https://doi.org/10.1080/08927014.2018.1425402

Rygiel K. (2018). Hypertriglyceridemia - Common Causes, Prevention and Treatment Strategies. *Current cardiology reviews, 14*(1), 67–76. https://doi.org/10.2174/1573403X14666180123165542

Saadi, M., & McCallum, R. W. (2013). Rifaximin in irritable bowel syndrome: rationale, evidence and clinical use. *Therapeutic advances in chronic disease, 4*(2), 71–75. https://doi.org/10.1177/2040622312472008

Saldivar, G. (2021, February 18). *How to Heal SIBO: The 3 Types.* 23 Nutrition Therapy -, MS RDN CLT IFNCP Functional Medicine Dietitian. Retrieved September 13, 2022, from https://www.23nutritiontherapy.com/how-to-heal-sibo-the-3-types/

Sanders, M. E. (2011, November). Impact of Probiotics on Colonizing Microbiota of the Gut. *Journal of Clinical Gastroenterology, 45*, S115–S119. https://doi.org/10.1097/mcg.0b013e318227414a

Samra, R. A. (2010). Fat Detection: Taste, Texture, and Post Ingestive Effects. (J. P. Montmayeur & J. le Coutre, Eds.). CRC Press/Taylor & Francis.

Sansone, R. A., & Sansone, L. A. (2010). Gratitude and well being: the benefits of appreciation. *Psychiatry (Edgmont (Pa. : Township)), 7*(11), 18–22.

Satokari R. (2020). High Intake of Sugar and the Balance between Pro- and Anti-Inflammatory Gut Bacteria. *Nutrients, 12*(5), 1348. https://doi.org/10.3390/nu12051348

Scazzocchio, B., Minghetti, L., & D'Archivio, M. (2020). Interaction between Gut Microbiota and Curcumin: A New Key of Understanding for the Health Effects of Curcumin. Nutrients, 12(9), 2499. https://doi.org/10.3390/nu12092499

Sender, R., Fuchs, S., & Milo, R. (2016). Revised Estimates for the Number of Human and Bacteria Cells in the Body. *PLoS biology, 14*(8), e1002533. https://doi.org/10.1371/journal.pbio.1002533

Shankle, W. R., & M.D., D. A. G. (2005). Preventing Alzheimer's: Ways to Help Prevent, Delay, Detect, and Even Halt Alzheimer's Disease and Other Forms of Memory Loss. In Preventing Alzheimer's: Ways to Help Prevent, Delay, Detect, and Even Halt Alzheimer's Disease and Other Forms of Memory Loss (pp. 5–299). TarcherPerigee.

Silván, J. M., Morales, F. J., & Saura-Calixto, F. (2010). Conceptual study on maillardized dietary fiber in coffee. *Journal of agricultural and food chemistry, 58*(23), 12244–12249. https://doi.org/10.1021/jf102489u

The Simplified Guide to the gut-brain axis - how the gut talks to the brain. Psych Scene Hub. (2021, October 27). Retrieved April 20, 2022, from https://

psychscenehub.com/psychinsights/the-simplified-guide-to-the-gut-brain-axis/

Simopoulos, A. (2006). Evolutionary aspects of diet, the omega-6/omega-3 ratio and genetic variation: nutritional implications for chronic diseases. *Biomedicine & Pharmacotherapy, 60*(9), 502–507. https://doi.org/10.1016/j.biopha.2006.07.080

Shao, Y., Forster, S. C., Tsaliki, E., Vervier, K., Strang, A., Simpson, N., Kumar, N., Stares, M. D., Rodger, A., Brocklehurst, P., Field, N., & Lawley, T. D. (2019). Stunted microbiota and opportunistic pathogen colonization in caesarean-section birth. *Nature, 574*(7776), 117–121. https://doi.org/10.1038/s41586-019-1560-1

Shreiner, A. B., Kao, J. Y., & Young, V. B. (2015). The gut microbiome in health and in disease. Current Opinion in Gastroenterology, 31(1), 69–75. https://doi.org/10.1097/mog.0000000000000139

the Society for Endocrinology. (2017, January). *Corticotrophin-releasing hormone.* You and your hormones. Retrieved April 20, 2022, from https://www.yourhormones.info/hormones/corticotrophin-releasing-hormone/

Small intestinal bacterial overgrowth (SIBO) - Symptoms and causes. (2022, January 6). Mayo Clinic. Retrieved September 5, 2022, from https://www.mayoclinic.org/diseases-conditions/small-intestinal-bacterial-overgrowth/symptoms-causes/syc-20370168

Smith, R. P., Easson, C., Lyle, S. M., Kapoor, R., Donnelly, C. P., Davidson, E. J., Parikh, E., Lopez, J. V., & Tartar, J. L. (2019). Gut microbiome diversity is associated with sleep physiology in humans. PLOS ONE, 14(10), e0222394. https://doi.org/10.1371/journal.pone.0222394

Stool Changes and What They Mean. (2019). Cleveland Clinic. https://my.clevelandclinic.org/health/articles/9663-stool-changes-and-what-they-mean

Sunrise Hospital & Medical Center. (2017). Being Healthy Starts in Your Gut: Tips for Promoting Optimal Gut Health and Preventing Disease. https://sunrisehospital.com/about/newsroom/being-healthy-starts-in-your-gut-tips- for-promoting-optimal-gut-health-and-preventing-disease

Takahashi T. (2012). Mechanism of interdigestive migrating motor complex. *Journal of neurogastroenterology and motility, 18*(3), 246–257. https://doi.org/10.5056/jnm.2012.18.3.246

Testing.(n.d.). SIBO - Small Intestine Bacterial Overgrowth. Retrieved September 9, 2022, from https://www.siboinfo.com/testing1.html

Tetel, M. J., de Vries, G. J., Melcangi, R. C., Panzica, G., & O'Mahony, S. M. (2018). Steroids, stress and the gut microbiome-brain axis. Journal of Neuroendocrinology, 30(2), e12548. https://doi.org/10.1111/jne.12548

Thaiss, C. A., Zeevi, D., Levy, M., Zilberman-Schapira, G., Suez, J., Tengeler, A. C., Abramson, L., Katz, M. N., Korem, T., Zmora, N., Kuperman, Y., Biton,

I., Gilad, S., Harmelin, A., Shapiro, H., Halpern, Z., Segal, E., & Elinav, E. (2014). Transkingdom control of microbiota diurnal oscillations promotes metabolic homeostasis. *Cell, 159*(3), 514–529. https://doi.org/10.1016/j.cell. 2014.09.048

Toro-Londono, M. A., Bedoya-Urrego, K., Garcia-Montoya, G. M., Galvan-Diaz, A. L., & Alzate, J. F. (2019). Intestinal parasitic infection alters bacterial gut microbiota in children. *PeerJ, 7*, e6200. https://doi.org/10.7717/peerj.6200

Tu, P., Chi, L., Bodnar, W., Zhang, Z., Gao, B., Bian, X., Stewart, J., Fry, R., & Lu, K. (2020). Gut Microbiome Toxicity: Connecting the Environment and Gut Microbiome-Associated Diseases. *Toxics, 8*(1), 19. https://doi.org/10.3390/toxics8010019

Uhde, M., Ajamian, M., Caio, G., De Giorgio, R., Indart, A., Green, P. H., Verna, E. C., Volta, U., & Alaedini, A. (2016). Intestinal cell damage and systemic immune activation in individuals reporting sensitivity to wheat in the absence of coeliac disease. Gut, 65(12), 1930–1937. https://doi.org/10.1136/gutjnl-2016-311964

van den Elsen, L., Garssen, J., Burcelin, R., & Verhasselt, V. (2019). Shaping the Gut Microbiota by Breastfeeding: The Gateway to Allergy Prevention?. Frontiers in pediatrics, 7, 47. https://doi.org/10.3389/fped.2019.00047

VanderWeele, T. J., & Brooks, A. C. (2020). A Public Health Approach to Negative News Media: The 3-to-1 Solution. *American Journal of Health Promotion.* https://doi.org/10.1177/0890117120914227

van Hoeken, D., & Hoek, H. W. (2020, August 17). Review of the burden of eating disorders: mortality, disability, costs, quality of life, and family burden. *Current Opinion in Psychiatry, 33*(6), 521–527. https://doi.org/10.1097/yco.0000000000000641

Weaver, K. R., Melkus, G. D., & Henderson, W. A. (2017). Irritable Bowel Syndrome. *The American journal of nursing, 117*(6), 48–55. https://doi.org/10.1097/01.NAJ.0000520253.57459.01

Weiss, E., & Katta, R. (2017). Diet and rosacea: the role of dietary change in the management of rosacea. *Dermatology practical & conceptual, 7*(4), 31–37. https://doi.org/10.5826/dpc.0704a08

Wellness Vision (2017 Five Common Medications Linked with Leaky Gut. https://www.wellnessvision.com.au/5-common-medications-cause-leaky-gut/

Wilkins, T., & Sequoia, J. (2018). Probiotics for Gastrointestinal Conditions: A Summary of the Evidence. *American Family Physician, 96*(3), 170–178. https://www.aafp.org/pubs/afp/issues/2017/0801/p170.html

Yang, Z., & Liao, S. F. (2019). Physiological Effects of Dietary Amino Acids on Gut Health and Functions of Swine. *Frontiers in veterinary science, 6,* 169 https://doi.org/10.3389/fvets.2019.00169

Zardast, M., Namakin, K., Esmaelian Kaho, J., & Hashemi, S. S. (2016). Assessment of antibacterial effect of garlic in patients infected with *Helicobacter pylori* using urease breath test. *Avicenna journal of phytomedicine, 6*(5), 495–501

Żukiewicz-Sobczak, W., Wróblewska, P., Adamczuk, P., & Silny, W. (2014). Probiotic lactic acid bacteria and their potential in the prevention and treatment of allergic diseases. *Central-European journal of immunology, 39*(1), 104–108. https://doi.org/10.5114/ceji.2014.42134

ABOUT THE AUTHOR

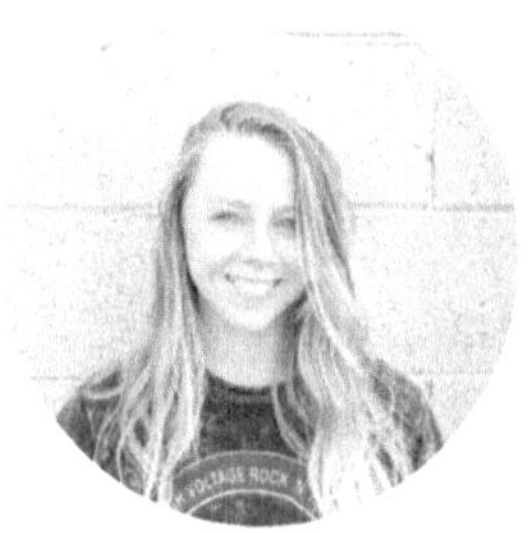

In 2018, Kara Holmes made her first chocolate donut with wholesome ingredients. She didn't want to feel deprived of delicious food while healing a gut and hormone imbalance. At the time, eating healthy seemed so out of reach—she was going on eleven years of disordered eating. But then something happened that she did not expect, and her effort to heal her gut helped her restore her relationship with food *and* release the weight her body no longer wanted. She left her career of eight years as a bedside registered nurse to make a deeper impact on the health of others, and the rest is history. When she isn't writing about how gut health can save your overall health, she is coaching others on gut healing and hormone nutrition, and creating delectable, anti-inflammatory recipes on her food blog. In her spare time, Kara enjoys a good sci-fi or fantasy flick, taking long hikes in nature to find hidden waterfalls, and exploring new cities.

Stay Connected and Up-to-Date

Follow me on my social media to get the latest gut health and hormone health tips, healthy dessert recipes, and healthy comfort food recipes.

YouTube: Kara Holmes @karaswellnessproject

Instagram: @karaswellnessproject

Tiktok: @karaswellnessproject

Questions? Email me at kara@vitalitycoaching.org